Alkaline Diet for Beginners 2020:

*222 Quick and Easy Recipes with
21 Day Meal Plan To
Improve Immune System
and Improve Digestion*

© Copyright July Anderson 2019 - All rights reserved.

The content contained within this book may not be reproduced, duplicated or transmitted without direct written permission from the author or the publisher.

Under no circumstances will any blame or legal responsibility be held against the publisher, or author, for any damages, reparation, or monetary loss due to the information contained within this book, either directly or indirectly.

Legal Notice:

This book is copyright protected. It is only for personal use. You cannot amend, distribute, sell, use, quote or paraphrase any part, or the content within this book, without the consent of the author or publisher.

Disclaimer Notice:

Please note the information contained within this document is for educational and entertainment purposes only. All effort has been executed to present accurate, up to date, reliable, complete information. No warranties of any kind are declared or implied. Readers acknowledge that the author is not engaging in the rendering of legal, financial, medical or professional advice. The content within this book has been derived from various sources. Please consult a licensed professional before attempting any techniques outlined in this book.

By reading this document, the reader agrees that under no circumstances is the author responsible for any losses, direct or indirect, that are incurred as a result of the use of information contained within this document, including, but not limited to, errors, omissions, or inaccuracies.

Table Of Contents

Introduction..5

Chapter 1 A Primer On The Alkaline Diet For Beginners 2020..................................6

Chapter 2 Alkaline Diet-Friendly Breakfast and Beverage Recipes.............18

Chapter 3 Alkaline Diet-Approved Lunch Recipes..51

Chapter 4 Alkaline Diet-Aligned Dinner Recipes..115

Chapter 5 Alkaline Diet-Accepted Snacks and Desserts...170

Conclusion...198

Introduction

This book has everything you need to adopt the alkaline diet in order to clear your body of harmful acids and give your immune system and digestive system a boost. It is teeming with many recipes – all 222 of them! – that lets you treat your palate while being mindful of your body's alkaline levels.

This book will help you feed your body with adequate nutrients, especially alkaline minerals, so that it is healed, energized, and able to optimally perform its functions. You can keep on enjoy eating healthy meals and snacks without sacrificing your body's health, and in return, you will be rewarded with an efficient immune system, better digestion, and a much improved state of health and well-being.

Thanks for downloading this book, I hope you enjoy it!

Chapter 1 A Primer On The Alkaline Diet For Beginners 2020

What It Means To Begin The Alkaline Diet In 2020

Moderation is what it is all about when following the alkaline diet lifestyle. Instead of depriving yourself of a specific food group, fixating on a particular "wonder" food item, or attempting to stick to an elaborate set of rules, the alkaline diet allows you to eat the foods you want in order to feed your body the proper nutrients for maintaining a health-promoting pH balance. The alkaline diet is scientifically built on the fact that your blood and body are intended to function optimally at a slightly alkaline pH level, which is 7.365. Your body's pH scale starts at 0 (highly acidic) and goes to 7 (neutral) and to 14 (pure alkaline). It helps to view this scale in terms of the good and the bad. Anything that is above 7 is alkaline and will do you good, and anything lower than 7 is acidic and not good for you. The fact is that your body has complex built-in control systems that ensure your pH level is stabilized, in the same way that your body will go to great lengths to keep your temperature regulated at 98.6 degrees Fahrenheit.

The Alkaline Connection Between Your Food and Your Body's Health

You may wonder why, if your body is already doing all it takes to maintain its pH at 7.365, you have to have to adopt an alkaline way of eating? The truth is that the purpose of following the alkaline diet is not to increase your body's alkalinity. Instead, it is about feeding your body plenty of alkaline minerals by consuming nutrient-dense foods like:

- fresh vegetables, organic leafy greens, and low-sugar fruits
- avocados and other healthy fats
- healthy whole grains
- nuts and seeds
- salads
- green drinks and smoothies

This way, your body does not have to use its own mineral reserves and compromise your health. Your body's pH can be brought down to an acidic level by acidic foods, which includes sugar, artificial sweeteners, dairy, gluten, processed foods, soda, alcohol, caffeinated drinks, and carbonated water, and they all cause your body to compensate by triggering a panic response, such as breathing in oxygen (alkaline) and exhaling carbon dioxide (acidic), urinating, and sweating.

In the same way that acid can burn through metal and leave a hole, acidic foods can do damage to your cardiovascular system, digestive system, and muscles and joints, and your body, as a form of defense mechanism, will try with all its might to keep that from taking place. This is why it will look for any possible sources of alkaline minerals to use in neutralizing the acids building up in your system, especially if the foods you eat are not supplying adequate minerals. Your body will inevitably cause damage to itself from robbing your muscles of magnesium (resulting in cramps and muscle pain), grabbing minerals from your teeth (causing tooth decay), and stripping your bones of calcium (leading to osteoporosis and joint pain). Your blood's pH level needs to be regulated, so much that your body will sacrifice itself to ensure that its pH does not stray from the ideal 7.365 mark.

How The Alkaline Diet Benefits Your Body's Well-Being

When you follow the alkaline diet, your body is not only able to keep its pH balance regulated and healthy, it is also equipped to energize as well as heal your body in several ways:

- *Supports good digestion*: The nutrients from the foods you eat are absorbed by your body through the numerous tiny folds (villi and microvilli) in your small intestine. But when you are clogged with acids, these folds get hidden, resulting in the blockage of your digestive system, reduced surface area of your small

intestine, and the inefficient absorption of nutrients. Eating alkaline foods will help you avoid this issue.
- *Gives your immune system a boost*: It is your immune system's main task to keep foreign invaders from attacking your body. But the presence of too much acid depletes oxygen, creating an environment that is hospitable to the growth of bacteria and viruses. Your immune system struggles to perform its function, causing you to be chronically prone to colds, flus, and even cancer. The alkaline diet can help reduce inflammation and oxygenate your cells, both of which promote a healthy immune system.
- *Maintains your muscle mass and bone density*: As suggested by research, eating more alkalizing vegetables and fruits can protect you from age-related muscle wasting as reduced bone strength. The alkaline diet balances the ratio of minerals needed to maintain muscle mass and build bones (calcium, phosphate, magnesium), as well as supports vitamin D absorption and growth hormone production, which provides added protection to your bones on top of alleviating other chronic diseases' effects.
- *Helps your body absorb vitamins and avoid suffering from magnesium deficiency*: Your body requires lots of magnesium in order to carry out numerous bodily processes and enable

many enzymes systems to function. When your magnesium levels go down, you can experience headaches, trouble with sleeping, muscle pains, heart complications, and feelings of anxiety.
- *Keeps your body at a healthy weight*: Even if the alkaline diet is not designed to aid in losing fat, adopting it in your lifestyle can result in weight loss as well as protect you from obesity. Eating less of foods that are acid-forming in the body and choosing to eat more of alkaline-forming foods results in reduced levels of leptin in your system, which helps reduce your hunger and improve your body's ability to burn fat and making it easier for you to shed off weight.
- *Reduces your chronic inflammation and pain*: Studies have shown that following an alkaline diet plan can help reduce chronic pain levels. It has also been found that suffering from chronic acidosis plays a role in chronic headaches, joint pain, back pain, muscle spasms, inflammation, and even menstrual symptoms.

Doing The Alkaline Diet in 2020 The Smart Way

Eating the alkaline way does not have to be complicated, especially with these handy tips and tricks to help you along the way:

1. Do food swaps

    Remove these from the pantry and fridge:
    - White rice and pasta
    - Granola and peanuts
    - Milk, milk chocolate, fruit juice, coffee, and bottled/tap water
    - Margarine, canola oil, balsamic vinegar, and soy sauce

    Have these better options:
    - Brown rice, oatmeal, and gluten-free pasta
    - Cashews and dark chocolate
    - Green tea, soy milk, fresh fruit juice, and filtered water
    - Butter and vegetable oil
    - Sea salt, brown sugar, apple cider vinegar, and wheat-free tamari

    Go for the best choices:
    - Spelt pasta, gluten-free quinoa, and gluten-free oats
    - Zucchini noodles
    - Lemon
    - Raw almonds and raw cacao
    - Green juices (cold-pressed), water with lemon, alkaline water, almond milk, coconut milk, and herbal tea

- Coconut oil, olive oil, avocado butter, and coconut butter
- Himalayan sea salt, Celtic sea salt, coconut sugar, stevia, and coconut aminos

2. Eat out smart
    - Choose to have salads, which are alkaline diet-friendly and help take the edge off hunger faster with their high water content.
    - Go for appetizers or side dishes instead of having a full entrée, and simply assemble them into a healthy meal.
    - When having fish or meat, have just a small portion, and have it steamed, baked, grilled, sautéed, roasted, or dehydrated.
    - Good to always have is an alkalizing soup with some sautéed brown rice or veggies.
    - Ask that all condiments and dressings be served on the side, or simply mix some fresh lemon juice with olive oil to make your own alkaline dressing.
    - Say no to soda and alcohol and down a glass of filtered/alkaline water with lemon instead.
    - Pass up on the bread.
    - It is good to have fresh fruit for dessert, better to share it with

everyone at the table, and best to skip it.

3. Give this 21-Day Alkaline Diet Meal Plan a try
   Starring some of the alkaline recipes featured in this book, this meal plan will help get you started on your alkaline eating journey.

21-Day Alkaline Diet Meal Plan

Day 1
Breakfast: Easy Avocado Toast
Lunch: Ginger Cauliflower Steaks
Snack: Carrot Cake Bites
Dinner: "Cheesy" Rotini Mushroom Casserole

Day 2
Breakfast: Almond Blueberry Quinoa
Lunch: Delectable Lemon Asparagus
Snack: Coconut Lime Pana Cotta
Dinner: Easy Spinach Pie

Day 3
Breakfast: Sunshine Burrito
Lunch: Apple and Butter Lettuce Salad
Snack: Mouthwatering Meltaway Balls
Dinner: Mock Beef Stew

Day 4
Breakfast: Overnight Banana Berry Breakfast Bowl
Lunch: Delicious Mexican Salad

Snack: Decadent Avocado Chocolate Pudding
Dinner: Potato Cakes with Green Peas Stuffing

Day 5
Breakfast: Tofu Scramble
Lunch: Green Peas and Melted Tomatoes
Snack: Spicy Herbed Flax Crackers
Dinner: Warm Cherry Tomatoes and Broccoli Salad

Day 6
Breakfast: Chia Flaxseed Pancakes
Lunch: Green Peas with Yellow Peppers
Snack: Green Pea Patties
Dinner: Veggie Primavera

Day 7
Breakfast: Scrumptious Sweet Potato Bowl
Lunch: Coriander and Tomatoes with Okra
Snack: Alkaline Granola Bars
Dinner: Zoodles Stuffed Tomatoes

Day 8
Breakfast: Carob Kamut Bars
Lunch: Mouthwatering Sesame Mixed Veggies
Snack: Green Peas Hummus
Dinner: Polenta with Asparagus and Mushroom Sauce

Day 9
Breakfast: Creamy Lime Avocado Smoothie
Lunch: Scrumptious Spinach with Almonds
Snack: Zucchini Flax Crackers
Dinner: Ancho Chili Chard Wrap

Day 10
Breakfast: Great Tasting Granola
Lunch: Lamb's Lettuce and Avocado Salad
Snack: Sweet Potato Brownies
Dinner: Amazing Aubergine Pizza

Day 11
Breakfast: Banana Spinach Smoothie
Lunch: Broccoli Sprouts and Green Cabbage Soup
Snack: Ginger Cookie Bites
Dinner: Sham Sushi

Day 12
Breakfast: Rosemary Carrot Soup
Lunch: Red Onion and Tomato Salad
Snack: Alkaline Energy Crackers
Dinner: Cherry Sea Veggies Salad

Day 13
Breakfast: Protein Bowl
Lunch: Collard Green and Carrot Burrito
Snack: Chocolate Pudding
Dinner: Delish Pesto Sweet Potato Casserole

Day 14
Breakfast: Creamy Lime Avocado Smoothie
Lunch: Basil Spinach Soup
Snack: Stuffed Peppers and Tomatoes
Dinner: Lime and Chipotle Cauliflower

Day 15
Breakfast: Easiest Breakfast Quinoa

Lunch: Bean Shoot and Broccoli Salad
Snack: Tasty Sweet Potato Chips
Dinner: Pineapple and Asian Kale Slaw

Day 16
Breakfast: Mouthwatering Almond Flour Pancakes
Lunch: Tasty Rocket Asparagus Salad
Snack: Easy Pickled Cucumbers
Dinner: Nutty Lemon and Apple Salad

Day 17
Breakfast: Choco Chia Pudding
Lunch: Crunchy Broccoli Sprouts Salad
Snack: Beetroot Ravioli Snack
Dinner: Avocado and Papaya Salad with Arugula

Day 18
Breakfast: Zucchini Chickpea Frittata
Lunch: Zesty Kale and Brussels Salad
Snack: Delicious Cinnamon Carrot Sticks
Dinner: Beet Kale and Red Kuri Salad

Day 19
Breakfast: Fenugreek Sprouts Breakfast Salad
Lunch: Avocado Quinoa Salad
Snack: Guacamole and Mushroom Bites
Dinner: Potatoes and Peas Stew

Day 20
Breakfast: Morning Pea Mash
Lunch: Sesame Lemongrass Tempeh Salad
Snack: Zucchini Chips

Dinner: Asian Style Mushrooms

<u>Day 21</u>
Breakfast: Tofu Avo Breakfast Salad
Lunch: Lemon Herb Zoodles
Snack: Spinach Power Balls
Dinner: Green Peas Ratatouille

Chapter 2 Alkaline Diet-Friendly Breakfast and Beverage Recipes

Sunshine Burrito
Ingredients:
Sauté:
Tempeh, steamed, pressed, diced (18 ounces)
Garlic clove, fresh (1 piece) or garlic powder (1 teaspoon)
Cayenne (1/8 teaspoon)
Black pepper (1/2 teaspoon)
Vegan butter (2 tablespoons)
Bell pepper, diced (3/4 cup)
Mushrooms, diced (1 cup)
Sweet onions (1/2 cup)
Turmeric (1 ½ teaspoons)
Sea salt, Himalayan pink (3/4 teaspoon)
Olive oil (1 teaspoon)
Apple cider vinegar (1 tablespoon)
Fold in:
Pepper jack cheese, Daiya (1/2 cup)
Spinach, organic, chopped (1 cup)
Coconut wraps, homemade (4 pieces)

Directions:
1. Heat vegan butter in pan to melt. Add onions, pepper, and mushrooms; sauté for two minutes.
2. Stir in tempeh, garlic, cayenne, bell pepper, sweet onion, turmeric, sea salt, olive oil, and apple cider vinegar. Saute

for five minutes, then add spinach, folding it in until wilted. Turn off heat before folding in the Daiya cheese as well.
3. Place wrap on a heated pan to warm. Top with the scrambled mixture, fold, and serve right away.

Easy Avocado Toast
Ingredients:
Bread slice, sprouted (1 piece)
Cherry tomatoes (1/2 cup)
Avocado, roughly mashed (1/2 piece)
Olive oil (1/2 teaspoon)
<u>Seasoning:</u>
Parsley
Sea salt

Directions:
1. Place avocado on bread slice.
2. Top with cherry tomatoes.
3. Drizzle all over with olive oil.
4. Season to taste.
5. Serve and enjoy.

Almond Blueberry Quinoa
Ingredients:
Quinoa, rinsed (1 cup)
Apple, medium, cubed (1 piece)
Stevia (1/4 teaspoon)
Almonds, raw, chopped (1/2 cup)
Sunflower seeds, raw (4 tablespoons)
Blueberries, organic, fresh (1 cup)

Almond milk, unsweetened (3 cups)
Vanilla (1/2 teaspoon)
Cinnamon (1 teaspoon)
Allspice (1/4 teaspoon)
Raisins (1/2 cup)
Toppings:
Raspberries/strawberries, fresh
Almonds, raw, chopped
Hemp seeds

Directions:
1. Mix together almond milk, raisins, quinoa, cinnamon, and allspice in a pan heated on medium. Let mixture boil, cover, and turn heat down to low. Cook for five minutes.
2. Add apple chunks and simmer for five minutes. Turn off heat and let sit for five minutes or until all the milk is absorbed.
3. Add stevia and top with desired toppings.

Tofu Avo Breakfast Salad
Ingredients:
Avocado, chopped (1 piece)
Pink grapefruit, chopped (1 piece)
Almonds, raw, chopped (1 handful)
Tortillas, heated in the oven, then baked for 10-min. (2 pieces)
Tofu, firm, chopped (1/2 pack)
Spinach, organic (4 handfuls)
Chili sauce (1 teaspoon)
Tomatoes, chopped (2 pieces)
Red onion, chopped (1/2 piece)

Lemon (1/2 piece)

Directions:
1. Toss chopped tomatoes, onions, and tofu with chili sauce. Let sit in the refrigerator for thirty minutes.
2. Toss the spinach along with the chopped avocado, grapefruit, and almonds.
3. Serve drizzled with lemon juice.

Fenugreek Sprouts Breakfast Salad
Ingredients:
Fenugreek sprouts, organic (1/2 cup)
Olive oil (2 tablespoons)
Herb mix, Italian (1/2 teaspoon)
Lime juice (1 teaspoon)
Red cabbage/radicchio (1/2 cup)
Radish, small, sliced thinly (1 piece)
Baby spinach/arugula, organic (1/2 cup)
Sea salt (1/4 teaspoon)
Black pepper, ground (1/4 teaspoon)

Directions:
1. Fill a large bowl with the sprouts and veggies. Toss to combine.
2. Mix olive oil and lime juice with sea salt, black pepper, and Italian herb mix. Add to veggie bowl and toss until well-coated.
3. Serve.

Morning Pea Mash
Ingredients:
Peas, boiled (1/2 cup)
Coconut oil (2 tablespoons)
Sea salt, Celtic (1/4 teaspoon)
Garlic, minced (3 tablespoons)
White onion, small (1 piece) or shallot (1 piece)
Kale, organic (1 bunch)

Directions:
1. Heat olive oil in a saucepan.
2. Add shallot and cook for two minutes.
3. Stir in minced garlic (1 tablespoon) and cook for one minute.
4. Add onion, minced garlic (2 tablespoons), and kale. Stir and cook for two minutes.
5. Stir in peas and cook for six minutes.
6. Add all other ingredients and cook for another two minutes.
7. Serve and enjoy.

Chia Flaxseed Pancakes
Ingredients:
Flax seed (1/4 cup)
Chia seeds (1/2 cup)
Seed flour (1/4 cup)
Sesame seed (1/4 cup)
Baking powder (1/2 teaspoon)
Sea salt, fine (1/4 teaspoon)
Stevia extract (1/2 teaspoon)
Buckwheat grouts (1 cup)
Cinnamon, ground (1 ½ teaspoons)
Almond milk

Coconut oil

Directions:
1. Combine seed flour with baking powder, sea salt, buckwheat grouts, cinnamon, and stevia.
2. Stir in sesame seeds, chia seeds, and flax seeds. Mix with just enough almond milk to make your batter.
3. Add coconut oil to a nonstick pan heated on medium. Gradually pour batter to form a thin layer. Cook until golden brown on both sides. Repeat with the rest of the batter.
4. Enjoy.

Overnight Banana Berry Breakfast Bowl
Ingredients:
Cinnamon (1/2 teaspoon)
Banana, sliced (1/2 piece)
Peanut butter (1/2 tablespoon)
Berries (1/2 cup)
Millet (1/2 cup)
Milk, skimmed (1/2 cup)
Yogurt (1/2 cup)

Directions:
1. Combine yogurt and millet with milk and sea salt inside a glass jar. Seal and let chill overnight.
2. Transfer in a serving bowl.
3. Top with berries and banana slices.
4. Enjoy.

Tofu Scramble
Ingredients:
Tofu (100 grams)
Paprika (1/2 teaspoon)
Yeast (1/2 cup)
Turmeric (1/2 teaspoon)
Baby spinach, organic (1/2 cup)
Onion, diced (1 piece)
Garlic cloves, minced (3 pieces)
Tomatoes (3 pieces)
Cumin (1/2 teaspoon)
Sea salt (1/4 teaspoon)
Coconut oil (1 tablespoon)

Directions:
1. Heat coconut oil in a pan heated on medium. Add onions and cook for five minutes. Stir in garlic and cook for one minute.
2. Toss in tomatoes and tofu. Cook for ten minutes.
3. Stir in paprika, cumin, and a little filtered/alkaline water. Cook for two minutes.
4. Stir in spinach and remove heat.
5. Serve right away.

Choco Chia Pudding
Ingredients:
Chia seeds (1/4 cup)
Cinnamon, ground (1/8 teaspoon)
Stevia extract (1/4 teaspoon)

Almond milk (1 ¼ cups)
Vanilla extract (1 teaspoon)
Cacao, raw, powdered (1 tablespoon)
Sea salt (1/8 teaspoon)

Directions:
1. Place all ingredients in a large bowl. Mix well.
2. Pour mixture into a mason jar. Refrigerate overnight.
3. Stir well and enjoy.

Mouthwatering Almond Flour Pancakes
Ingredients:
Almond butter (2 tablespoons)
Honey, raw (1 teaspoon)
Baking soda (1/8 teaspoon)
Almond flour (1 cup)
Cassava flour (1/2 cup)
Almond milk (1 ¼ cups)
Coconut oil (1 teaspoon)

Directions:
1. Stir the flours together in a large bowl. Add baking soda.
2. Combine all wet ingredients. Add to the flour mixture and mix well.
3. Add coconut oil to a skillet heated on medium.
4. Add batter, ¼ cup at a time. Cook for twp minutes on each side.
5. Serve topped with fruit.

Zucchini Chickpea Frittata
Ingredients:
Spring onions, chopped (1/2 cup)
Black pepper (1/2 teaspoon)
Olive oil (4 tablespoons)
Garlic, grated (1 clove)
Chickpea flour (1 cup)
Filtered/alkaline water (1 cup)
Zucchini slices (1 cup)
Onion, chopped (1/2 cup)
Sea salt (1/4 teaspoon)

Directions:
1. Set oven at 375 degrees Fahrenheit to preheat.
2. Mist cooking spray onto a baking tray.
3. Mix all ingredients in a bowl, save for the spring onions and oil. Stir in oil (2 tablespoons).
4. Pour mixture onto baking tray. Bake for thirty to forty-five minutes.
5. Slice frittata into serving portions and serve garnished with spring onions.

Carob Kamut Bars
Ingredients:
Vanilla (1 teaspoon)
Almond milk, unsweetened (1/2 cup)
Trail mix (1/2 cup + 2 tablespoons)
Kamut, whole grain, puffed (1 bag)
Mini marshmallows, vegan (2 bags)
Carob chips (1 cup)

Protein powder, vegan, vanilla flavored (2 scoops)

Directions:
1. Fill a large bowl with kamut. Set aside.
2. Combine almond milk and vanilla.
3. Mist cooking spray onto 2 baking pans.
4. Pour protein powder and almond milk into a pot. Heat on medium-high until boiling, stirring constantly.
5. Turn off heat before stirring in marshmallows. Once melted, pour mixture into kamut bowl. Gently toss in carob chips.
6. Add ¾ of the trail mix (1/2 cup) and mix well. Spread mixture onto greased pans. Top with remaining carob chips and trail mix (2 tablespoons), pressing down to make sure they stick.
7. Freeze for an hour.
8. Slice into 16 bars and serve.

Scrumptious Sweet Potato Bowl
Ingredients:
Sweet potatoes, mashed (1 cup) or sweet potato puree (8 ounces)
Pumpkin seeds (3 tablespoons)
Sesame seeds (2 teaspoons)
Olive oil (1/2 tablespoon)
Garlic, minced (2 teaspoons)
Spinach, organic (2 cups)

Directions:
1. Add oil to a skillet heated on medium.
2. Stir in garlic and cook for one minute.
3. Stir in spinach and cook for another one minute.
4. Add sweet potatoes to a saucepan heated on medium and cook until warned through.
5. Add spinach on top of sweet potatoes. Season with pepper and sea salt, then garnish with sesame seeds and pumpkin seeds.
6. Enjoy.

Creamy Lime Avocado Smoothie
Ingredients:
Tofu, natural silken (1/2 cup)
Lime, large, peeled (1 piece)
Stevia extract (1/4 teaspoon)
Ice (1/2 cup)
Cucumber, skin-on (3/4 cup)
Spinach, organic (3 cups)
Broccoli, organic, frozen (2 cups)
Avocado, medium (1/2 piece)
Almond milk, unsweetened (1/2 cup)

Directions:
1. Fill blender with all ingredients.
2. Process until creamy and smooth.
3. Serve and enjoy.

Rosemary Carrot Soup
Ingredients:
Parsley, fresh (1 cup)
Rosemary, dried (1 teaspoon)
Vegetable stock powder, yeast-free (25 teaspoons)
Cauliflower, chopped (2 cups)
Onion, large (1 piece)
Celery stick (3 pieces)
Carrots, large (3 pieces)
Garlic cloves (5 pieces)
Green broccoli sprouts, organic, chopped (3 cups)
Sea salt (1/2 teaspoon)
Pepper, cracked (1/4 teaspoon)
Filtered/alkaline water, filtered (2 liters)

Directions:
1. Fill a pressure cooker with all ingredients.
2. Cover and cook for thirty minutes.
3. Pour into a serving bowl.
4. Enjoy with brown rice.

Easiest Breakfast Quinoa
Ingredients:
Almond milk (1 ½ cups)
Filtered/alkaline water (1/2 cup)
Quinoa (1/2 cup)
Cinnamon (1/4 teaspoon)
Vanilla extract (1 teaspoon)
Coconut oil (1 tablespoon)

Directions:
1. Pour quinoa into a saucepan heated on medium.
2. Cook for two to three minutes, stirring constantly.
3. Stir vanilla, filtered/alkaline water, and almond milk into the toasted quinoa.
4. Let mixture boil, then reduce heat to medium-low.
5. Simmer for twenty-five minutes, stirring constantly.

Banana Spinach Smoothie
Ingredients:
Flaxseeds/chia seeds (1 tablespoon)
Almond butter (1 tablespoon)
Ice cubes (3 pieces)
Filtered/alkaline water /almond milk (1 cup)
Banana, ripe (1 piece)
Spinach, organic (2 handfuls)

Directions:
1. Place all ingredients in the blender.
2. Process until well-combined and smooth.
3. Serve and enjoy.

Great Tasting Granola
Ingredients:
Currants/cranberries/goji, dried (1/2 cup)
Filtered/alkaline water (2 tablespoons)
Coconut oil (3 tablespoons)
Brown rice syrup (1/3 cup)

Almonds, raw (2 cups)
Pine nuts, raw (2 cups)
Pumpkin seeds, raw (1 cup)
Coconut, shredded, unsweetened (1 cup)
Vanilla extract (1 teaspoon)
Cinnamon, ground (1/2 teaspoon)
Himalayan sea salt (1/2 teaspoon)

Directions:
1. Set oven at 300 degrees Fahrenheit to preheat.
2. Use parchment paper in lining a baking sheet.
3. Roughly chop up the pine nuts, pumpkin seeds, and almonds in the blender.
4. Whisk coconut oil, filtered/alkaline water, brown rice syrup, cinnamon, sea salt, and vanilla in a large bowl.
5. Combine the dry mixture with the wet mixture. Spread evenly on lined baking sheet and bake for twenty minutes, shuffling halfway.
6. Remove from the oven and let cool for ten minutes.
7. Enjoy.

Protein Bowl
Ingredients:
Capsicum, sliced (1/2 piece)
Broccoli florets, steamed (1 handful)
Avocado, cubed (1 piece)
Quinoa, uncooked (50 grams)
Spinach leaves, organic, sliced (1 handful)

Kale leaves, sliced (1 handful)
Flax oil
Cherry tomatoes, halved (12 pieces) or tomatoes, large, halved (2 pieces)
Lemon juice (2 teaspoons)
Himalayan sea salt (1/4 teaspoon)
Black pepper (1/4 teaspoon)

Directions:
1. Follow package directions in cooking the quinoa.
2. Toss everything inside a large bowl.
3. Serve drizzled with lemon juice and flax oil.

Vanilla Ginger Porridge
Ingredients:
Nutmeg, freshly ground (1/2 teaspoon)
Coconut cream/milk (1/2 cup)
Lemon peel, grated (1 teaspoon)
Vanilla bean pod (1 piece)
Quinoa, dry (1 cup)
Filtered/alkaline water (2 cups)
Cinnamon stick (1 piece)
Ginger, freshly grated (1 ½ teaspoons)
Assorted seeds & nuts, raw (1/2 handful)
Toppings:
Cloves, ground
Coconut yogurt

Directions:
1. Follow package directions in cooking the quinoa. Drain and return to the pan.

2. Add the spices, vanilla, and coconut cream/milk. Stir and cook until creamy and thick.
3. Serve topped with coconut yogurt, ground cloves, grated lemon peel, and extra cinnamon.

Creamy Coco Chia Pot

Ingredients:
Coconut yogurt (1 cup)
Flax meal (1 tablespoon) or flax seeds, ground (1 tablespoon)
Sesame seeds (1 teaspoon)
Coconut milk, organic (1 cup)
Chia seeds (1/4 cup)
Date (1 piece)
Vanilla extract (1/2 teaspoon)

Directions:
1. Process the dates and coconut milk in the blender until well-blended. Pour into a large bowl.
2. Stir in vanilla, sesame seeds, chia seeds, and flaxmeal. Refrigerate for thirty minutes.
3. Place coconut yogurt (1/2 cup) in a small glass. Top with chia mixture and finish by adding the remaining coconut yogurt (1/2 cup).

Berry Blueberry Smoothie
Ingredients:
Flax seeds, ground (1 tablespoon)
Coconut milk (1 cup)
Coconut oil (1 tablespoon)
Hemp seed powder (1 tablespoon)
Blueberries (1/2 cup)
Almond butter, raw (1 tablespoon)
Spinach, organic (1 handful)
Chia seeds (1 tablespoon)

Directions:
1. Process all ingredients in the blender until well-combined.
2. Pour into a tall glass.
3. Enjoy.

Pumpkin and Buckwheat Pancakes
Ingredients:
Allspice (1/4 teaspoon)
Nutmeg (1/4 teaspoon)
Cinnamon (1/2 teaspoon)
Butternut squash/pumpkin, medium, chopped, steamed (1/2 piece)
Buckwheat flour (1 ½ cups)
Sea salt (1/2 teaspoon)
Ginger (1/2 teaspoon)
Flax seeds, ground (2 tablespoons)
Brown rice syrup (2 tablespoons)
Almond milk (2 cups)
Coconut oil (2 tablespoons)
Lemon juice (1/2 teaspoon) + baking soda (1/4 teaspoon)

Coconut yogurt – to serve

Directions:
1. Process the pumpkin chunks and coconut oil in the blender until smooth.
2. Mix lemon juice (1/2 teaspoon) with baking soda (1/4 teaspoon) inside a large bowl. Whisk in spices, sea salt, and buckwheat flour.
3. In a separate bowl, whisk together the pumpkin, almond milk, flax, and brown rice syrup. Pour pumpkin mixture into the buckwheat mixture and whisk well to combine.
4. Add coconut oil to a large saucepan heated on medium-low. Working in batches, add batter and cook until golden brown on both sides.
5. Serve pancakes topped with coconut yogurt.

Easy Breakfast Bars
Ingredients:
Brown rice syrup (3 tablespoons)
Ginger, 1-inch, grated (1 piece) or ginger, ground (2 teaspoons)
Coconut oil (2 tablespoons)
Millet, uncooked (5 cups)
Almond butter (320 grams)
Coconut cream (1 cup)

Directions:
1. Fill a large bowl with coconut oil, brown rice syrup, and coconut cream. Whisk well to combine.
2. Whisk in ginger and almond butter.
3. Add the millet and mix well.
4. Place millet mixture in a parchment-lined baking dish and spread to form an even layer.
5. Refrigerate overnight.
6. Slice into bars and serve.

Cashew Cucumber Smoothie
Ingredients:
Pine nuts, raw (1 handful)
Oats, organic (1 handful)
Coconut milk (250 milliliters)
Filtered/alkaline water, filtered (200 milliliters)
Coconut oil (1 tablespoon)
Almonds, raw (1 handful)
Chia seeds (1 handful)
Avocado (1/2 piece)
Cucumber (1 piece)
Kale/baby spinach leaves, organic (1 handful)

Directions:
1. Fill blender with chia seeds and liquid ingredients. Let sit for two minutes.
2. Add the rest of the ingredients.
3. Process until smooth.
4. Serve and enjoy.

Vanilla Bircher and Coconut Pots
Ingredients:
Vanilla broccoli sprouts, organic, ground (1 teaspoon) or vanilla paste (1 teaspoon)
Flax meal (1 tablespoon)
Almond milk (1 cup)
Date, chopped (1 piece)
Millet (1 cup)
Coconut oil (1 tablespoon)
Chia seeds (1 tablespoon)
Coconut, shredded (1 tablespoon)
Pumpkin seeds (1 tablespoon)
Sunflower seeds (1 tablespoon)
Cinnamon (1 pinch)
Himalayan sea salt (1 pinch)

Directions:
1. Stir all ingredients together inside a mason jar.
2. Refrigerate overnight.
3. Serve.

Avocado Spinach Bowl
Ingredients:
Kale/beet greens, organic (2 handfuls)
Baby spinach, organic (4 handfuls)
Avocado, large, roughly chopped (1 piece)
Sea salt (1/4 teaspoon)
Pepper, cracked (1/4 teaspoon)
Sweet potato, large, sliced thinly (1 piece)
Coconut oil (2 tablespoons)
Garlic cloves, chopped finely (2 pieces)
Broccoli florets, organic (8 pieces)

Sunflower seeds (1 tablespoon)
Chia seeds (1 tablespoon)
<u>Dressing:</u>
Lemon juice (180 milliliters)
Ginger, freshly grated (2 teaspoons)
Black pepper, cracked (1/4 teaspoon)
Himalayan sea salt (1/4 teaspoon)
Coconut aminos, homemade (4 tablespoons)
Filtered/alkaline water (4 tablespoons)
Olive oil/flax (2 tablespoons)

Directions:
1. Set the oven at 400 degrees Fahrenheit to preheat.
2. Coat sweet potato slices with half of coconut oil. Bake for fifteen to twenty minutes.
3. Process dressing ingredients in the blender until smooth.
4. Add remaining coconut oil to a skillet heated on medium. Add garlic; after one minute, add broccoli, kale/beet greens, and baby spinach. Stir and cook for five minutes.
5. Place sweet potatoes on a plate lined with paper towels.
6. Line individual bowls with drained sweet potatoes, then fill with veggies and seeds. Top with dressing and serve.

Almond Breakfast Smoothie
Ingredients:
Coconut oil (1 tablespoon)
Chia seeds (1 tablespoon)
Almond butter (1 tablesploon)
Avocado (1/2 piece)
Baby spinach leaves, organic (2 handfuls)
Kale/watercress, organic (2 handfuls)
Almonds, raw, soaked overnight (1/2 cup)
Almond milk, unsweetened (200 milliliters)
Filtered/alkaline water (200 milliliters)

Directions:
1. Process all ingredients, except the chia seeds, in the blender.
2. Pour mixture into a tall glass.
3. Stir in chia seeds. Let sit for two minutes.
4. Serve and enjoy.

Buckwheat Sesame Seed Pancakes
Ingredients:
Buckwheat flour (1 cup)
Baking soda (1 ½ teaspoons)
Himalayan sea salt (1 teaspoon)
Stevia (1/4 teaspoon)
Pumpkin seeds (1/4 cup)
Flax seeds (1/2 cup)
Sunflower seeds (1/4 cup)
Sesame seeds (1/4 cup)
Milk, soy/almond
Oil, olive/coconut

Directions:
1. Grind the seeds in the coffee grinder. Place ¼ of mixture in a large bowl (save the rest for other use). Add buckwheat flour, stevia, sea salt, and baking soda. Mix well before stirring in soy/almond milk.
2. Heat a nonstick skillet on medium. Add coconut oil.
3. Working in batches, pour batter and cook pancakes until golden on both sides.

Apple Quinoa Breakfast Warmer
Ingredients:
Coconut oil (1 tablespoon)
Quinoa (1/2 cup)
Apple (1 piece)
Lemon (1/2 piece)
Cinnamon
Optional:
Nuts, raw
Seeds, raw
Cranberries, dried

Directions:
1. Follow package directions in cooking the quinoa.
2. Add the rest of the ingredients to the cooked quinoa. Stir until well-combined.
3. Serve sprinkled with cinnamon and enjoy.

Delicious Baked Broccoli Sprouts Brekkie
Ingredients:
Spinach, organic (2 handfuls)
Garlic cloves (2 pieces)
Avocado, halved, pitted (1 piece)
Lemon (1/2 piece)
Broccoli sprouts, organic (15 ounces)
Spring onions (4 pieces)
Cherry tomatoes (6 pieces)
Basil (1 handful)
Coconut oil (1 teaspoon)
Black pepper
Himalayan sea salt
Olive oil

Directions:
1. Chop up all veggies.
2. Heat a saucepan on medium. Add garlic and a little water; stir and cook for one minute.
3. Stir in spring onions, cherry tomatoes, and broccoli sprouts. Cook for five minutes.
4. Stir in coconut oil, spinach, basil, black pepper, and sea salt. Cook for ten minutes.
5. Drizzle with olive oil and lemon juice before serving with halved avocado.

Coconut Cinnamon Breakfast Parfait
Ingredients:
Cardamom, ground (1 pinch)
Himalayan sea salt (1 pinch)

Chia seeds, soaked for 2 minutes (2 tablespoons)
Mixed berries, organic (120 grams)
Coconut, shredded, unsweetened (40 grams)
Coconut oil (2 tablespoons)
Cinnamon, ground (1 pinch)
Coconut yogurt (200 milliliters)
Coconut cream, canned (200 milliliters)

Directions:
1. Set oven at 300 degrees Fahrenheit to preheat.
2. Combine shredded coconut with sea salt and spices. Stir in coconut oil before transferring to a parchment-lined sheet. Bake for five minutes, then let cool.
3. Fill wide glasses with layered fruit, coconut cream, and chia seeds. Top with coconut mixture and coconut yogurt. Serve garnished with fruit.

Heavenly Bread
Ingredients:
Millet (1 cup)
Flax seeds (3 tablespoons)
Flour, coconut/buckwheat (1/2 cup)
Chia seeds (3 tablespoons)
Sunflower seeds (1/2 cup)
Pumpkin seeds (1/4 cup)
Almonds, raw (1/2 cup)
Psyllium husks (4 tablespoons)
Coconut oil, melted (3 tablespoons)
Almond butter (1 tablespoon)
Coconut flakes (4 tablespoons)

Filtered/alkaline water (400 milliliters)

Directions:
1. Combine all dry ingredients inside a large bowl.
2. Combine all wet ingredients in another bowl.
3. Add the wet mixture to the dry mixture and combine into a doughy mixture. Let stand for two to three hours.
4. Set oven at 350 degrees Fahrenheit to preheat.
5. Press dough into a loaf tin. Bake for twenty minutes, flip bread upside down, and bake for an additional twenty minutes.
6. Let cool before serving.

Vanilla Almond Cookies
Ingredients:
Medjool dates, pitted (6 pieces)
Vanilla (1 teaspoon)
Vanilla bean, split, w/ seeds removed (1 piece)
Filtered/alkaline water (2 tablespoons + more as needed)
Almonds, raw (1 cup)
Millet (1/2 cup)
Almond butter (3 tablespoons)
Stevia, pure (3 tablespoons)
Sea salt (1 pinch)
Cacao, raw (1/4 cup)
Optional:
Cinnamon (1/2 teaspoon)

Coconut flakes (1/4 cup)

Directions:
1. Process all ingredients, except the chocolate chips, in the blender until well-combined. Transfer to a large bowl and stir in chocolate chips.
2. Let sit in the fridge for twenty minutes.
3. Mold into cookie shapes. Sprinkle with cinnamon and/or coconut flakes.
4. Serve and enjoy.

Chili Chai Hot Choco

Ingredients:
Cardamom powder (1 teaspoon)
Cinnamon powder (1 teaspoon)
Red chili (1 piece)
Coconut oil (1 tablespoon)
Coconut/almond milk (450 milliliters)
Root ginger, 1-inch, sliced (1 piece)
Almond butter (1 tablespoon)
Cacao, raw (2 tablespoons)

Directions:
1. Slice the ginger before adding to a skillet heated on medium-low.
2. Stir in oil, almond butter, milk, raw cacao, and spices.
3. Simmer for five to ten minutes. Pour into the blender and process until smooth and frothy.
4. Serve sprinkled with cinnamon.

Turmeric Tea
Ingredients:
Almond/coconut milk (500 milliliters)
Cinnamon (1 teaspoon)
Turmeric, 1-inch, freshly sliced (1 piece)
Ginger, 1-inch, freshly sliced (1 piece)
Coconut oil (1 tablespoon)
Maca powder (1 teaspoon)
Brown rice syrup (1 teaspoon)

Directions:
1. Slice ginger and turmeric before adding to a saucepan filled with coconut oil, brown rice syrup, milk, maca powder, and cinnamon. Heat on medium-low and simmer for five minutes.
2. Turn off heat and let mixture sit for ten minutes.
3. Pour mixture into the blender and process until frothy and well-blended.
4. Serve right away.

Energizing Kale Smoothie
Ingredients:
Swiss chard, organic (3 handfuls)
Almonds, raw (25 pieces)
Pumpkin seeds (1 handful)
Avocado (1 piece)
Kale, organic (3 handfuls)
Cucumber, small (1 piece)
Spinach, organic (4 handfuls)
Broccoli sprouts, organic (1/2 cup)
Water, filtered/alkaline (200 milliliters)

Directions:
1. Add all ingredients to a blender.
2. Process until everything is well-blended.
3. Serve right away.

Nourishing Beetroot Juice
Ingredients:
Ginger, ½-inch (1 piece)
Turmeric, 1-inch (1 piece)
Beetroot (1 piece)
Carrot (1 piece)
Cucumber (1 piece)
Kale, organic (1/2 bunch)
Spinach, organic (2 handfuls)
Grapefruit (1/2 piece)

Directions:
1. Place all ingredients, except the grapefruit, in the food processor.
2. Blitz until you have a smooth mixture.
3. Serve and enjoy.

Skinny Spinach Juice
Ingredients:
Beetroot, medium, w/ leaves (1 piece)
Cucumber (1 piece)
Baby spinach, organic (3 handfuls)
Kale, organic (1/2 bunch)
Cinnamon (1/2 teaspoon)

Directions:
1. Place all ingredients, except the cinnamon, in the blender.
2. Process until everything is evenly combined.
3. Stir in cinnamon and serve immediately.

Soothing Ginger Tonic
Ingredients:
Thyme leaves & stalk, fresh (2 teaspoons)
Sage leaves, fresh (2 teaspoons)
Filtered/alkaline water (1 liter)
Lemon (1 piece)
Ginger root, fresh, 2-cm (1 piece)
Turmeric root, 1-cm (1 piece)

Directions:
1. Heat water to boiling, then let simmer before adding lemon zest and lemon juice.
2. Stir in the rest of the ingredients.
3. Cook on simmer for five minutes.
4. Let cool for one minute before straining.
5. Serve and enjoy.

Super Creamy Almond Chia Smoothie
Ingredients:
Nutmeg (1 teaspoon)
Rooibos tea, loose leaf (10 grams)
Almonds, raw (2 handfuls)
Coconut oil (1 tablespoon)
Coconut cream (250 milliliters)
Ginger root, ½-inch (1 piece)

Cinnamon (1 teaspoon)
Cardamom (1 teaspoon)
Chia seeds (1 tablespoon)
Almond milk, unsweetened (250 milliliters)
Avocado (1/2 piece)
Optional:
Vanilla pod (1 piece)
Watercress/kale (1 handful)

Directions:
1. Heat a saucepan on medium-low.
2. Pour in almond milk and coconut milk. Stir in rooibos tea leaves, ginger root, cardamom, cinnamon, and nutmeg.
3. Cook on a simmer for five minutes. Strain into a blender.
4. Add cooked ginger root, chia seeds, almonds, coconut oil, and avocado. Process until well-blended and smooth.
5. Serve immediately.

Chocolate Coconut Smoothie
Ingredients:
Coconut yogurt (3 tablespoon)
Coconut oil (3 teaspoons)
Raw cacao (3 tablespoons)
Maca powder (1 tablespoon)
Avocado, ripe (1/2 piece)
Spinach, organic (2 handfuls)
Almond milk (200 milliliters)
Coconut milk (200 milliliters)
Almonds, raw, soaked (50 grams)
Pine nuts, raw (25 grams)

Sunflower seeds (1 tablespoon)
Chia seeds (1 tablespoon)

Directions:
1. Process everything in the blender until smooth.
2. Pour into a tall glass.
3. Enjoy.

Cucumber and Celery Juice
Ingredients:
Ginger, raw, 1/2 –inch (1 piece)
Turmeric, raw, ½-inch (1 piece)
Lemon juice (2 teaspoons)
Tomatoes (2 pieces)
Celery stalk (1 piece)
Garlic clove (1 piece)
Cucumber (1 piece)

Directions:
1. Add all ingredients to the blender.
2. Process until evenly combined.
3. Serve right away.

Refreshing Cucumber Juice
Ingredients:
Cucumbers (2 pieces)
Lemon juice, fresh (4 tablespoons)
Celery (1/2 head)
Kale/spinach, organic (5 ounces)
Turmeric root (1 tablespoon)

Directions:
1. Blend all ingredients in the food processor.
2. Strain into a glass.
3. Enjoy.

Chapter 3 Alkaline Diet-Approved Lunch Recipes

Lemon Herb Zoodles
Ingredients:
Dill sprig leaves, fresh (1 pinch)
Cilantro/parsley sprig tops, fresh (1 pinch)
Garlic powder (1 dash)
Onion (1 dash)
Zucchini noodles, raw (1 cup)
Hemp hearts (1/2 cup)
Lemon juice (1 tablespoon)
Chives, chopped (1 teaspoon)
Himalayan sea salt (1/4 teaspoon)
Filtered/alkaline water (1/3 cup + more as needed)

Directions:
1. Process all ingredients in the blender until smooth.
2. Add on top of zucchini noodles.
3. Serve and enjoy.

Sesame Lemongrass Tempeh Salad
Ingredients:
Lime juice, fresh (1 teaspoon)
Mint, chopped (1 tablespoon)
Coriander, chopped (1 tablespoon)
Spring onions, chopped (2 pieces)
Lemongrass stalks, minced (2 pieces)
Sesame seeds, toasted (2 teaspoons)
Pine nuts, raw (1 handful)

Asian shallots, small, thinly sliced (5 pieces)
Garlic cloves, thinly sliced (2 pieces)
Lime, fresh – for garnishing
Vegetable oil - for frying
Tempeh:
Sriracha (1 teaspoon)
Almond flour (1 tablespoon)
Tempeh, cubed (3/4 cup)
Tamarind concentrate, wheat-free (1 ½ teaspoons)

Directions:
1. Toss all salad ingredients in a large bowl. Set aside.
2. Add oil (1/2 inch) to a skillet heated on medium. Stir in pine nuts and cook for half a minute; immediately place on a plate lined with paper towels. Repeat with the garlic.
3. Toss tempeh ingredients in a large bowl. Add to the same oil in skillet and cook until fried through. Transfer to a plate lined with paper towels.
4. Add tempeh mixture to the salad and serve right away.

Avocado Quinoa Salad
Ingredients:
Quinoa (1 ½ cups)
Pine nuts, raw (1/2 cup)
Olive oil, extra virgin (1/4 cup)
Lemon juice, fresh (3 tablespoons)
Cucumber, peeled, diced (1 piece)

Avocado, w/ stone removed, quartered (1 piece)
Roma tomatoes, seeded, chopped finely (3 pieces)
Red onion, small, chopped finely (1 piece)
Lemon zest, grated (2 teaspoons)
Parsley, fresh, chopped (1 handful)
Himalayan sea salt (1/4 teaspoon)
Black pepper, freshly ground (1/4 teaspoon)

Directions:
1. In a large pot, heat 2 liters of alkaline/filtered water to boiling. Add quinoa, then turn heat down to medium-low. Cover and cook for fifteen minutes.
2. Set oven at 390 degrees Fahrenheit to preheat.
3. Place pine nuts on baking tray and toast in oven for three to four minutes. Let cool before adding to a large bowl.
4. Drain and rinse the cooked quinoa before adding to the pine nuts. Stir in parsley, onion, cucumber, and tomatoes.
5. Season mixture with pepper and sea salt. Sprinkle with lemon juice, lemon zest, and olive oil before garnishing with avocado.
6. Serve salad right away.

Zesty Kale and Brussels Salad
Ingredients:
Pomegranate seeds (2 tablespoons)
Himalayan pink sea salt (1/4 teaspoon)
Black pepper, coarsely ground (1/4 teaspoon)

Tuscan kale leaves, sliced into thin strips (2 bunches)
Brussels sprouts, organic, sliced finely (15 pieces)
Almonds, raw, chopped roughly (1/3 cup)
Pine nuts, raw (2 tablespoons)
<u>Dressing:</u>
Molasses (1 teaspoon)
Olive oil (1/4 cup)
Mint leaves, chopped finely (8 pieces)
Shallots, minced (1 tablespoon)
Garlic cloves, minced (2 pieces)
Coconut aminos (2 tablespoons)
Lemon juice freshly squeezed (1/4 cup)

Directions:
1. Whisk all salad dressing ingredients together until well-blended.
2. Place remaining ingredients in a large bowl. Toss to combine.
3. Add dressing to salad bowl and toss until evenly mixed.
4. Serve immediately.

Crunchy Broccoli Sprouts Salad
Ingredients:
Broccoli sprouts, organic (1/2 cup)
Almonds, raw, chopped roughly (2 tablespoons)
Pine nuts, raw (1 tablespoon)
Pumpkin seeds (1 tablespoon)
Kale, organic, w/ stalks removed, sliced roughly (4 handfuls)
Brussels sprouts, organic, thinly shaved (8 pieces)

Radishes, sliced thinly (2 pieces)
Carrot, sliced thinly (1 piece)
Basil, chopped (1 cup)
Dressing:
Flax/olive oil (1 tablespoon)
Lemon juice, fresh (2 tablespoons)
Black pepper, cracked (1/4 teaspoon)
Avocado, large (1/2 piece)
Coconut aminos (1 tablespoon)
Garlic clove (1 piece)
Himalayan sea salt (1 pinch)

Directions:
1. Toss all salad ingredients together.
2. Add dressing ingredients to a blender. Process until smooth.
3. Pour dressing over salad and toss gently.
4. Enjoy.

Tasty Rocket Asparagus Salad
Ingredients:
Tuscan kale, organic, sliced (2 handfuls)
Rocket, organic (2 handfuls)
Asparagus, sliced (1 bunch)
Lemon juice (1 teaspoon)
English cucumber, sliced (1 piece)
Sea salt (1/4 teaspoon)
Pepper, cracked (1/4 teaspoon)
Dressing:
Coconut aminos (1 teaspoon)
Shallot, diced finely (1/4 piece)
Lemon juice (1/4 cup)
Olive oil (1/2 cup)

Directions:
1. Combine all dressing ingredients.
2. Mix all salad ingredients together.
3. Toss salad with the dressing. Season with pepper and sea salt.
4. Serve and enjoy.

Spelt Fettucini
Ingredients:
Rosemary, fresh, chopped (1 ½ teaspoons)
Almond milk, unsweetened (1/4 cup)
Lemon juice, fresh (1 tablespoon)
Celtic sea salt (1 tablespoon + ¼ teaspoon)
Spelt fettuccini noodles, cooked (4 cups)
Garlic cloves, halved (10 pieces)
Olive oil, extra virgin (1/4 cup + 3 tablespoons)
Broccoli sprouts, organic, drained, rinsed, steamed (14 ounces)
Green peas, fresh, sliced lengthwise, halved, steamed (1 pound)
Asparagus spears, halved, steamed (1 bunch)
Red peppers, sliced into quarter-inch strips, steamed (2 pieces)
Pistachio topping:
Pistachios, raw, lightly toasted (1/2 cup)
Lemon zest, grated finely (1 tablespoon)
Sea salt, fine (1/8 teaspoon0
Chili flakes (1/4 teaspoon)

Directions:
1. Combine all pistachio topping ingredients. Set aside.

2. Heat a saucepan on medium. Add olive oil (2 tablespoons) and garlic. Cook for five minutes, then let cool.
3. Place green peas, olive oil (1/4 cup), lemon juice, sea salt (1/4 teaspoon), and rosemary in the blender. Add sautéed garlic and almond milk and process until smooth.
4. Drain cooked fettuccini and gently toss with steamed veggies and prepared sauce.
5. Serve topped with crushed pistachios.
6. Enjoy.

Bean Shoot and Broccoli Salad
Ingredients:
Salad:
Cucumber, large, peeled, seeded, sliced into matchsticks (1 piece)
Coriander, fresh, finely chopped (2 cups)
Green onions, finely sliced (1 bunch)
Carrots, shredded (3 cups)
Broccoli stalks, sliced into matchsticks (2 cups)
Mung bean shoots (2 cups)
Dressing:
Garlic clove, crushed (1 piece)
Red chili, deseeded (1 piece)
Lime juice, freshly squeezed (1/2 cup)
Sesame oil (3 tablespoons)
Garnish:
Almonds, raw, chopped
Sesame seeds

Directions:
1. Process all dressing ingredients, except the garlic and chili, in the blender until smooth. Stir in chili and garlic.
2. Mix all salad ingredients.
3. Toss salad with the dressing.
4. Serve garnished with raw almonds or sesame seeds.

Easy Peasy Salad
Ingredients:
Peas, fresh, roughly chopped (400 grams)
Green asparagus, lightly steamed, chopped (100 grams)
Green pepper, roughly chopped (1 piece)
Spring onions, roughly chopped (2 pieces)
Spinach leaves, organic, fresh, chopped (1 bag)
Tomatoes, sliced (3 pieces)
Dressing:
Olive oil (1 tablespoon)
Himalayan sea salt (1/4 teaspoon)
Avocado (1 piece)
Lemon juice, fresh (1 tablespoon)

Directions:
1. Mash avocado with other dressing ingredients until well-blended.
2. Place the remaining salad ingredients in a large bowl.
3. Gently toss salad with the dressing.
4. Season with sea salt before serving.

Basil Spinach Soup
Ingredients:
Celery stalk (1 piece)
Avocado (1/4 cup)
Tomato, chopped (1/2 piece)
Olive oil (2 tablespoons)
Spinach, organic, chopped (1/2 bunch)
Basil, loose (1 cup)
Red onion, chopped (1/4 cup)
Cucumber, medium (1/2 piece)
Garlic clove, medium (1/2 piece)
Celtic sea salt (1/2 teaspoon)
Pine nuts, raw (1/4 cup)

Directions:
1. Process everything in the blender.
2. Pour into a pot and heat on medium.
3. Once warmed through, pour soup into serving bowl.
4. Serve garnished with tomatoes and drizzled with olive oil.

Watercress and Cucumber Soup
Ingredients:
Lemon, freshly squeezed (2 pieces)
Watercress, organic (1 ½ cups)
Sea salt (1/4 teaspoon)
Pepper (1/4 teaspoon)
Haas avocados, organic (3 pieces)
Scallions (2 pieces)
Cucumber, diced (1 cup)
Filtered/alkaline water (2 cups)
Cherry tomatoes, halved (1/4 cup)

Directions:
1. Put everything in the blender.
2. Process until pureed into a smooth mixture.
3. Season with pepper and sea salt.
4. Serve with cherry tomatoes on top.

Collard Green and Carrot Burrito
Ingredients:
Collard green, organic, w/ stem removed (1 piece)
Cucumber, sliced into matchsticks (1/2 piece)
Carrot, sliced into matchsticks (1 piece)
Haas avocado, sliced (1/2 piece)
Mung bean sprouts, organic (1 handful)
Basil, chopped (2 sprigs)
Mint, chopped (4 sprigs)
Cilantro, chopped (1 handful)
<u>Dipping sauce:</u>
Green onion, sliced (1 piece)
Tamari, gluten-free (1/4 cup)
Ginger, minced (1 teaspoon)
Garlic clove, minced (1 piece)

Directions:
1. Combine all dipping sauce ingredients.
2. Roll the collard green and stuff with all other ingredients.
3. Serve burrito and dipping sauce right away.

Avocado Dressed Grapefruit and Watercress Salad

Ingredients:
Salad:
Sour grapefruit, sliced into sections (1 piece)
Almonds, raw, sliced (1/2 cup)
Watercress, organic (2 cups)
Broccoli florets, organic (2 cups)
Dressing:
Chia seeds (1/2 tablespoon)
Sea salt (1/4 teaspoon)
Black pepper (1/4 teaspoon)
Haas avocado, medium (1/2 piece)
Coconut oil (2 tablespoons)
Apple cider vinegar (1 tablespoon)

Directions:
1. Mix all salad ingredients in a large bowl.
2. Blend all dressing ingredients in the blender.
3. Gently toss the salad with the dressing.
4. Season to taste, serve, and enjoy.

Red Onion and Tomato Salad

Ingredients:
Olive oil, extra virgin (2 tablespoons)
Lime juice, freshly squeezed (1 tablespoon)
Cumin (1 teaspoon)
Pepper (1/4 teaspoon)
Celtic sea salt (1/4 teaspoon)
Haas avocados, diced (2 pieces)
Red onion, diced (1/2 piece)
Tomato, diced (1 piece)

Cilantro/parsley, fresh, chopped finely (1/4 cup)
Jalapeno, diced (1/4 piece)

Directions:
1. Season avocado pieces with pepper and sea salt.
2. Mix tomatoes with onion, cumin, and cilantro. Season to taste before placing on top of avocados.
3. Toss everything with jalapeno, lime juice, and olive oil.

Broccoli Sprouts and Green Cabbage Soup
Ingredients:
Green cabbage, organic, chopped (100 grams)
Spinach, organic, chopped (100 grams)
Rucola, organic, chopped (50 grams)
Rosemary twigs, chopped (2 pieces)
Olive oil (4 tablespoons)
Vegetable stock, yeast-free (1 liter)
Green peas, steamed (15 ounces)
Carrot, julienned (1 piece)
Celery stick, minced (1 piece)
Garlic cloves, minced (2 pieces)
Pumpkin bread, alkaline-friendly, day-old (60 grams), cubed – *see Chapter 1 for* **Pumpkin Bread** *recipe*
Red onion, minced (1 piece)
Himalayan sea salt (1 pinch)
Black pepper, freshly ground (1 pinch)

Directions:
1. Add oil (1 tablespoon) to a large pot heated on medium-high. Stir in garlic, celery, and carrot. Cook for one minute, then add rosemary and remaining vegetables. Cook for ten minutes.
2. Stir in bread pieces and stock. Cook for two minutes, then turn heat down to medium. Cover and cook for fifteen minutes.
3. Season with pepper and sea salt and serve immediately.

Lamb's Lettuce and Avocado Salad
Ingredients:
Salad:
Carrots, grated (2 pieces)
Almonds, raw (10 pieces)
Spinach, organic, fresh (2 handfuls)
Lamb's lettuce, organic (2 handfuls)
Pepper, freshly ground (1/4 teaspoon)
Himalayan sea salt (1/4 teaspoon)
Dressing:
Avocado, large (1 piece)
Tomato (1 piece)
Onion, small (1 piece)
Garlic clove, small (1 piece)
Olive oil, extra virgin (2 tablespoons)
Lime juice, freshly squeezed (1 tablespoon)

Directions:
1. Mix up all salad ingredients in a large bowl.

2. Combine all dressing ingredients before adding to salad bowl. Gently toss until everything is well-mixed.
3. Season to taste and serve immediately.

Scrumptious Spinach with Almonds
Ingredients:
Coconut oil (8 tablespoons)
Almonds, raw, skinned (80 grams)
Red chili, dried, crumbled (1 piece)
Curry powder (1 teaspoon)
Spinach, organic, fresh, torn (600 grams)
Onion, small, minced (1 piece)
Garlic clove, minced (1 piece)
Tomato, ripe, diced (1 piece)
Coriander, ground (1/2 teaspoon)
Celtic sea salt (1 pinch)

Directions:
1. Add oil to a frying pan heated on medium-high. Stir in almonds and chili and cook for two minutes. Transfer to a plate lined with paper towels.
2. Add garlic and onion to same pan and cook for two minutes. Stir in coriander, curry powder, and tomato. Cook for two minutes.
3. Stir in spinach and cook for two minutes before adding almonds and sea salt.
4. Serve and enjoy.

Mouthwatering Sesame Mixed Veggies

Ingredients:
Celery sticks, julienned, steamed (4 pieces)
Rape seed oil (3 tablespoons)
Celtic sea salt (1/4 teaspoon)
Pepper, freshly ground (1/4 teaspoon)
Sesame seeds, peeled, roasted (50 grams)
Carrots, julienned, steamed (400 grams)
Broccoli, organic, chopped, steamed (700 grams)
Leeks, chopped (300 grams)

Directions:
1. Add oil to a wok heated on medium-high.
2. Stir in all veggies and cook for five minutes.
3. Season with pepper and sea salt.
4. Serve garnished with sesame seeds.

Coriander and Tomatoes with Okra
Ingredients:
Coriander seeds, crushed (2 teaspoons)
Garlic cloves, crushed (3 pieces)
Lemon rind, grated finely (1 teaspoon)
Lemon juice, freshly squeezed (1 teaspoon)
Himalayan sea salt (1/4 teaspoon)
Black pepper, ground (1/4 teaspoon)
Tomatoes, ripe, chopped (450 grams)
Okra, fresh, trimmed (450 grams)
Olive oil (3 tablespoons)
Onions, sliced thinly (2 pieces)

Directions:
1. Add oil to a frying pan heated on medium. Stir in onions and coriander to cook for three to four minutes.
2. Stir in garlic and okra and cook for one minute. Add tomatoes and cook on a simmer for twenty minutes.
3. Stir lemon juice, lemon zest, pepper, and sea salt into the dish before serving.

Green Peas with Yellow Peppers
Ingredients:
Green peas, steamed (250 grams)
Thyme, dried (1 teaspoon)
Vegetable stock (400 milliliters)
Spring onions, sliced into rings (4 pieces)
Onions, minced (2 pieces)
Garlic cloves, minced (2 pieces)
Yellow peppers, sliced (350 grams)
Olive oil (2 tablespoons)
Sea salt (1/4 teaspoon)
Pepper, freshly ground (1/4 teaspoon)
Lemon juice, fresh (1 ½ tablespoons)

Directions:
1. Heat pot on medium after adding oil. Stir in garlic and onions. Cook for two minutes before stirring in green peas, yellow peppers, vegetable stock, and thyme. Let mixture boil, then cover and cook on a simmer for ten minutes.
2. Add spring onion rings, cover, and cook for another two minutes.

3. Sprinkle with peppers, sea salt, and lemon juice before serving.

Tofu and Tomato Scramble
Ingredients:
Rocket/arugula, organic (1 handful)
Brown onion (1/2 piece), minced
Red pepper, small, diced (1/2 piece)
Turmeric (1 pinch)
Tofu, firm, crumbled (285 grams)
Coconut oil (1 tablespoon)
Tomatoes, diced (2 pieces)
Baby spinach, organic (2 handfuls)
Black pepper, freshly ground (1/4 teaspoon)
Himalayan sea salt (1/4 teaspoon)
Basil (1 pinch)
Cilantro/coriander (1 pinch)
Cayenne pepper (1 pinch)

Directions:
1. Add onion to a skillet heated on medium and filled with a little coconut oil. Cook for two minutes.
2. Stir in diced red pepper and cook for another two minutes.
3. Add tomatoes, spinach, tofu, sea salt, pepper, and turmeric. Cook for ten minutes.
4. Toss in remaining veggies and cook for five minutes.
5. Serve and enjoy.

Delicious Mexican Salad
Ingredients:
Almonds, raw, chopped (1 handful)
Baby spinach, organic, chopped (4 handfuls)
Chili sauce (1 tablespoon)
Lettuce leaves, organic (2 pieces)
Tofu, firm (1/2 pack)
Avocado, sliced (1 piece)
Pink grapefruit, sliced (1 piece)
Tomatoes (2 pieces)
Red onion (1/2 piece)
Lemon (1/2 piece)

Directions:
1. Set oven at 350 degrees Fahrenheit to preheat.
2. Set lettuce leaves over the bottom side of a medium-sized bowl. Bake for two minutes or until crisp and bowl-shaped. Set aside to cool.
3. Chop up the tomatoes, tofu, and onion. Combine with chili sauce and refrigerate for ten minutes.
4. Toss everything together in a large bowl. Serve topped with spinach and drizzled with lemon juice.

Apple and Butter Lettuce Salad
Ingredients:
Salad:
Beet, small, spiralized (1 piece)
Purple cabbage, organic, chopped (1 cup)
Hemp seeds (2 tablespoons)

Butter lettuce, organic, chopped (1 head)
Green apple, spiralized (1 piece)
Sunflower seeds (2 tablespoons)
Dressing:
Olive oil, extra virgin (2/3 cup)
Cilantro, chopped (1/4 cup)
Lemon juice, fresh (1/4 cup)
Apple cider vinegar (2 tablespoons)
Black pepper (1 teaspoon)
Sea salt (1/4 teaspoon)

Directions:
1. Combine all salad ingredients in a large bowl.
2. Whisk together the ingredients for the dressing.
3. Add dressing to the salad bowl. Toss until evenly coated.
4. Serve and enjoy.

Avocado Salad with Pumpkin Seeds
Ingredients:
Coconut aminos (3 teaspoons)
Kale, organic, chopped (2 bunches)
Coconut oil (2 tablespoons)
Avocados, chopped (3 pieces)
Pumpkin seeds (1/4 cup)

Directions:
1. Add oil to a saucepan heated on medium-high.
2. Stir in kale and cook for five minutes.

3. Stir in coconut aminos before topping with pumpkin seeds and avocado.

Garlic Green Broccoli Sprouts
Ingredients:
Green broccoli sprouts, organic (1 ½ pounds)
Red pepper flakes (2 teaspoons)
Sea salt (1/4 teaspoon)
Coconut oil (2 tablespoons)
Garlic cloves (5 pieces)

Directions:
1. Add oil to a skillet heated on medium-high.
2. Stir in garlic and cook for two minutes.
3. Stir in broccoli, sea salt, and chili flakes. Cover and cook for five minutes.
4. Serve right away.

Delectable Lemon Asparagus
Ingredients:
Garlic, minced (2 cloves)
Lemon juice, fresh (1 teaspoon)
Asparagus (1 bunch)
White onion, chopped (1/4 piece)
Olive oil
Pepper
Sea salt

Directions:
1. Set oven at 350 degrees Fahrenheit to preheat.

2. Line a glass baking dish with asparagus. Top with remaining ingredients and cover with foil.
3. Bake for thirty minutes.
4. Serve immediately.

Ginger Cauliflower Steaks

Ingredients:

Cauliflower, organic, sliced into ¾-inch-thick "steaks" (1 head)
Himalayan sea salt (1/4 teaspoon)
Pepper (1/4 teaspoon)
Coconut oil (1 tablespoon)
Sauce:
Cumin, ground (1 teaspoon)
Turmeric, ground (1/2 teaspoon)
Olive oil, extra virgin (1 tablespoon)
Ginger, freshly grated (1 teaspoon)
Cilantro, chopped (1 tablespoon)

Directions:

1. Set oven at 400 degrees Fahrenheit to preheat.
2. Add coconut oil to a skillet heated on medium. Season cauliflower steaks with pepper and sea salt, then add to the pan. Cook for two minutes on each side.
3. Whisk together olive oil, turmeric, ginger, and cumin.
4. Transfer cauliflower steaks to a parchment-lined baking sheet. Brush with ginger mixture before roasting for fifteen minutes.

5. Serve garnished with cilantro.

Watermelon and Cucumber Salad
Ingredients:
Olive oil, extra virgin (1 tablespoon)
Lime juice, fresh (2 tablespoons)
Avocados, sliced (2 pieces)
Cucumbers, peeled, cubed (2 pieces)
Tomato, diced (1 piece)
Cilantro, chopped (1/3 cup)
Black pepper (1/4 teaspoon)
Sea salt (1/4 teaspoon)
Arugula (1 handful)

Directions:
1. Mix avocado with lime juice and olive oil.
2. Toss remaining ingredients in a large bowl. Top with avocado mixture.
3. Serve and enjoy.

Red Bell Pepper Quinoa and Mixed Greens Salad
Ingredients:
Mixed greens, organic (1 handful)
Bell pepper, red, chopped (1 cup)
Avocado (1 piece)
Beet, shredded (1 piece)
Tomato, large (1 piece)
Carrot, shredded (1 piece)
Cucumber, chopped (1 piece)
Dressing:
Garlic clove (1 piece)

Lemon juice (1 ½ tablespoons)
Apple cider vinegar (2 ½ tablespoons)
Sea salt (1 ½ teaspoons)
Bell pepper, red, chopped (1 ½ cups)
Carrot, chopped (1/4 cup)
Ginger (1 ½ tablespoons)
Olive oil (1/2 cup)
Filtered/alkaline water (as needed)
Quinoa:
Quinoa (1 cup)
Boiling water, filtered/alkaline (1 ½ cups)

Directions:
1. Mix all ingredients for the dressing.
2. Toss all salad ingredients. Top with prepared dressing.
3. Enjoy.

Lemon and Avocado Dressed Kale Salad
Ingredients:
Lemon juice (1/2 cup)
Olive oil (1/3 cup)
Avocado, mashed (1 piece)
Dinosaur kale leaves, organic (5 pieces)
Red onion, chopped (1/2 piece)
Garlic cloves, chopped (2 pieces)
Sea salt (1/4 teaspoon)

Directions:
1. In a large bowl, mash the avocado, olive oil, and lemon juice until well-blended.
2. Toss in kale leaves and remaining ingredients.

3. Serve right away.

Romaine Lettuce Wraps with Walnut Hummus Spread

Ingredients:
Tomato, small (1 piece)
Basil, fresh, chopped (1 teaspoon)
Broccoli sprouts, organic, cooked after getting soaked overnight (1/4 cup)
Romaine lettuce leaves, organic (3 pieces)
Avocado, mashed (1 piece)
Cucumber, chopped (1/2 piece)
<u>Almond hummus:</u>
Almonds, raw, dry, soaked in warm filtered/alkaline water for 2 hrs (1 1/8 cups)
Himalayan sea salt (1 1/8 teaspoons)
Cayenne (1/4 teaspoon)
Paprika (1 ½ teaspoons)
Zucchini, chopped (2 cups)
Garlic cloves (2 pieces)
Olive oil (3 tablespoons)
Lemon juice (1/4 cup)
Cumin (1 teaspoon)
Filtered/alkaline water (1 tablespoon)
Coconut aminos (1/4 cup)

Directions:
1. Mash avocado and spread on lettuce leaves.
2. Combine ingredients for almond hummus spread and add on top of avocado spread.
3. Top with remaining ingredients and season to taste.

4. Wrap, serve, and enjoy.

Cumin Cauli Rice
Ingredients:
Lemon zest (1 tablespoon)
Cumin (2 teaspoons)
Stevia (2 teaspoons)
Ginger, freshly grated (1 teaspoon)
Cauliflower head, organic, medium (1 piece)
Peas, fresh (1 cup)
Scallions, sliced thinly (4 pieces)
Lemon juice, fresh (1/2 cup)
Pine nuts, raw (1/2 cup)
Chili flakes (1 tablespoon)
Pepper (1/4 teaspoon)
Himalayan sea salt (1/4 teaspoon)

Directions:
1. Process cauliflower in the blender until rice like in texture.
2. Place cauliflower in a large bowl filled with peas and scallions.
3. Add a mixture of lemon juice, stevia, cumin, ginger, and lemon zest.
4. Toss until everything is well-combined.
5. Season to taste and serve topped with chili flakes and pine nuts.

Warming Quinoa and Vegetable Soup
Ingredients:
Broccolini stalks, chopped (6 pieces)
Leeks, chopped (3 ½ ounces)

Lime juice (2 tablespoons)
Tamari, wheat-free (2 teaspoons)
Quinoa, cooked (1 cup)
Vegetable bouillon powder, yeast-free (1 ½ teaspoons)
Filtered/alkaline water (1 ¾ cups + 1 cup)
Cilantro, chopped (4 tablespoons)

Directions:
1. Fill a pot with one cup of water (alkaline/filtered).
2. Add leeks, tamari, lime juice, and broccolini.
3. Cook on a simmer for five minutes.
4. Stir in quinoa.
5. Serve garnished with cilantro.

Walnut Taco Salad
Ingredients:
Taco meat:
Cumin powder (1/2 teaspoon)
Sea salt, fine (1/4 teaspoon)
Almonds, raw, soaked for 8 hrs (1/2 cup)
Chili powder (1 ½ teaspoons)
Cayenne pepper (1/4 teaspoon)
Cream sauce:
Macadamia nuts, soaked for 8 hrs (1 cup)
Himalayan sea salt, fine (1/3 teaspoon)
Filtered/alkaline water (12 tablespoons)
Lemon juice, fresh (2 tablespoons)
Guacamole:
Cumin, ground (1/2 teaspoon)
Lime juice, fresh (1 tablespoon + 1 teaspoon)

Sea salt, fine (1/4 teaspoon)
Avocado, ripe, large (1 piece)
Red onion, chopped (1/4 cup)
Tomato, small, chopped (1/2 piece)
Other salad ingredients:
Mixed greens, organic
Green onion
Salsa

Directions:
1. Process taco meat ingredients in the blender until slightly chunky. Set aside.
2. Process cream sauce in the blender until smooth.
3. Mash avocado before mixing with other guacamole ingredients.
4. Fill a large bowl with mixed greens. Add guacamole (1/4 cup), salsa (2 tablespoons), and taco meat (1/2 portion) on top.
5. Finish by smothering with cream sauce and garnishing with green onion.

Fennel Mushroom Salad
Ingredients:
Olive oil (2 tablespoons)
Fennel, diced (3 ¼ ounces)
Lemon juice (2 teaspoons)
Pumpkin seeds, raw (1/2 tablespoon)
Portobello mushroom (1 piece)
Garlic cloves, chopped finely (2 pieces)
Thyme sprigs (3 pieces)
Himalayan sea salt (1 pinch)

Parsley, flat leaf, chopped roughly (1/4 ounces)

Directions:
1. Set oven at 350 degrees Fahrenheit to preheat.
2. Spread mushrooms on baking sheet. Top with sea salt, thyme, garlic, and olive oil.
3. Bake for fifteen minutes.
4. Toss fennel with lemon juice and olive oil. Add on top of mushroom salad.
5. Serve sprinkled with parsley and pumpkin seeds.

Tasty Pasta Primavera
Ingredients:
Bell pepper, yellow, sliced thinly into strips (1 piece)
Bell pepper, red, sliced thinly into strips (1 piece)
Olive oil, cold-pressed (1/4 cup)
Sea salt (1/4 teaspoon)
Pepper (1/4 teaspoon)
Carrots, peeled, sliced thinly into strips (3 pieces)
Zucchini, medium, sliced thinly into strips (2 pieces)
Yellow squash, sliced thinly into squash (2 pieces)
Onions, sliced thinly (1 piece)
Italian seasoning (1/4 cup)
Basil, chopped (1/4 cup)
Cherry tomatoes, chopped (1/2 cup)
Spaghetti squash (1 cup)

Directions:
1. Spread all vegetables on baking sheet. Toss with olive oil, pepper, dried Italian herbs, and sea salt. Bake for twenty minutes.
2. Add zucchini and toss to combine. Bake for another thirty minutes.
3. Serve topped with cherry tomatoes and basil.

Green Peas and Melted Tomatoes
Ingredients:
Coconut oil, extra virgin (1 tablespoon)
Tomato, diced (1 cup)
Ginger, freshly grated (1 teaspoon)
Tomatoes, sundried, olive oil-packed, diced finely (4 pieces)
Green peas (1/2 cup)
Vegetable broth, yeast-free (1 ½ cups)
Shallot/white onion, minced (1/3 cup)
Garlic cloves, minced (3 pieces)
Filtered/alkaline water (4 tablespoons)
Spinach, organic, fresh, chopped (2 cups)
Baby kale, organic, chopped (2 cups)
Himalayan sea salt (1/4 teaspoon)
Pepper, freshly ground (1/4 teaspoon)
Olive oil, extra virgin (1 tablespoon)

Directions:
1. Fill a pot with vegetable broth and green peas. Heat to boiling, then cook on simmer for twenty minutes.

2. Saute garlic and onions in a skillet heated on medium-low for two minutes. Stir in tomatoes and alkaline/filtered water (2 tablespoons) and cook for another two minutes. Stir in ginger, chopped greens, and additional alkaline/filtered water (2 tablespoons) and cook for two minutes. Stir in the green peas.
3. Serve seasoned with pepper and sea salt and drizzled with olive oil.

It's A Wrap!
Ingredients:
Sweet pickles, chopped finely (2 tablespoons)
Dill, fresh, chopped finely (2 tablespoons)
Parsley, fresh, chopped finely (2 tablespoons)
Dulse flakes (1 ½ tablespoons)
Sunflower seeds, raw, soaked overnight while refrigerated (1 ½ cups)
Olive oil (1 ½ tablespoons)
Sea salt (1/2 teaspoon)
Celery, chopped finely (1/4 cup)
Lemon juice (1 tablespoon)
Romaine lettuce wrap, organic

Directions:
1. Process sunflower seeds, sea salt, and olive oil in the blender until chunky and pasty.
2. Combine sunflower paste with remaining ingredients.
3. Fill romaine lettuce wrap with mixture.
4. Serve and enjoy.

Yummy Butternut Squash Risotto
Ingredients:
Hot filtered/alkaline water (2 ½ cups)
Vegetable stock, yeast-free (2 cups)
Sage leaves, chopped (1 handful)
Himalayan sea salt (1 pinch)
Butternut squash, sliced (7 ounces)
Olive oil (3 tablespoons)
Red onion, chopped (1 piece)
Risotto rice, brown (5/6 cup)

Directions:
1. Set oven at 350 degrees Fahrenheit to preheat.
2. Spread squash pieces on baking sheet and drizzle with olive oil (2 tablespoons). Bake for fifteen minutes.
3. Add remaining oil to a pan heated on medium. Stir in garlic and onions. After two minutes, stir in rice and cook for two minutes.
4. Pour in vegetable stock, 2 ladlefuls at a time, and simmer until mixture absorbs half of the vegetable stock.
5. Stir in sage leaves and butternut squash. Add remaining stock and simmer for fifty minutes or until all liquid is absorbed.
6. Serve right away.

Easy Cauliflower Fried Rice
Ingredients:
Zucchini, sliced thinly (1 piece)

Ginger, ½-inch, fresh, grated (1 piece)
Turmeric, ½-inch, fresh, grated (1 piece)
Cauliflower, organic, large, grated into rice-like texture (1 piece)
Kale, organic, sliced thinly (1/2 bunch)
Coconut oil (1 tablespoon)
Lime juice (1 tablespoon)
Spring onions, chopped (4 pieces)
Almonds, raw, chopped (2 handfuls)
Coriander, chopped (1 bunch)
Parsley, chopped (1/2 bunch)
Mint, chopped (1 bunch)
Coconut aminos (1 tablespoon)
Pepper, ground (/4 teaspoon)
Sea salt (1/4 teaspoon)

Directions:
1. Heat a large pan filled with coconut oil. Stir in mint, parsley, and coriander. Cook for half a minute before adding the cauliflower and kale. Cook for three minutes.
2. Stir in coconut aminos, spring onions, and remaining herbs. Turn off heat after two minutes.
3. Season with pepper and sea salt and drizzle with lime juice.
4. Serve topped with chopped almonds.

Ginger Asparagus Broth
Ingredients:
Garlic cloves, minced (2 pieces)
Red chili, fresh, chopped (1 piece)

Asparagus stalks, chopped (8 pieces)
Kale, organic, chopped (1 handful)
Vegetable stock, gluten-free (3 cups)
Filtered/alkaline water (2 cups)
Tamari, gluten-free (1 ½ tablespoons)
Root ginger, 1-inch, fresh, peeled, grated (1 piece)
Spring onion, chopped (1 piece)
Coconut oil (1 tablespoon)
Black pepper, cracked (1/4 teaspoon)
Himalayan sea salt (1/4 teaspoon)
Coriander, fresh, chopped (1/2 cup)
Olive oil (1 glug)

Directions:
1. Add coconut oil, water, vegetable stock, and tamari to a saucepan heated on medium. Mix well.
2. Stir in chili, ginger, and garlic. Cook on a simmer for four minutes.
3. Add the asparagus, kale, coriander, and spring onion.
4. Place in serving bowl and drizzle on top with olive oil.

Turmeric Cauliflower Salad
Ingredients:
Avocado, cubed (1/2 piece)
Tomatoes, cubed (2 pieces)
Turmeric, fresh, grated (2 tablespoons)
Cayenne pepper (1/4 teaspoon)
Cauliflower head, organic, washed, rinsed, dried, chopped into florets (1/2 piece)

Curly kale stalks, organic, washed, rinsed, chopped (5 pieces)
Bell pepper/capsicum, sliced (1 piece)
Celery stalk, sliced (1 piece)
Tamari, wheat-free (1/4 teaspoon)
Himalayan sea salt (1/4 teaspoon)
Black pepper (1/4 teaspoon)
Paprika (1/4 teaspoon)
Lemon (1/2 piece)
Pumpkin seeds
Olive oil
Coconut oil

Directions:
1. Set oven at 355 degrees Fahrenheit to preheat.
2. Toss cauliflower florets with coconut oil (2 tablespoons), paprika, turmeric, sea salt, pepper, and cayenne pepper.
3. Spread mixture on a parchment-lined baking tray. Bake for twenty minutes.
4. Toss kale with lemon juice and tamari. Transfer to serving plate. Top with avocado, tomato, bell pepper, and celery. Sprinkle with olive oil and sesame seeds.
5. Top salad with cauliflower and enjoy.

Minty Summer Salad
Ingredients:
Radish, sliced thinly (5 pieces)
Green peas, cooked (200 grams)
Zucchini, sliced thinly (2 pieces)
Avocado, sliced (1 piece)

Asparagus, blanched, sliced into strips (3 bunches)
Cilantro, chopped roughly (1/2 bunch)
Parsley, flat leaf, chopped roughly (1/2 bunch)
Dressing:
Garlic clove, crushed (1 piece)
Olive oil (190 milliliters)
Coconut aminos (15 grams)
Lemon juice (3 tablespoons)
Shallots, diced (2 pieces)
Mint, chopped roughly (1/4 bunch)
Black pepper (1/4 teaspoon)
Himalayan sea salt (1/4 teaspoon)

Directions:
1. Brown zucchini in pan heated on medium.
2. Add zucchini to a large bowl filled with remaining veggies. Toss to combine.
3. Mix all dressing ingredients in the blender. Add to the salad and gently toss until evenly coated.
4. Season to taste before serving.
5. Enjoy.

Hearty Tomato and Chickpea Soup
Ingredients (cooked):
Broccoli head, organic (1/4 piece)
Green cabbage head, organic (1/4 piece)
Vegetable stock (200 milliliters)
Tomatoes, fresh, chopped (8 pieces)
Brown onion, roughly sliced (1 piece)
Garlic cloves, roughly chopped (2 pieces)
Carrots, sliced (2 pieces)

Cauliflower head, organic (1/4 piece)
Himalayan pink sea salt (1/4 teaspoon)
Black pepper (1/4 teaspoon)
Ginger root, ½-inch (1 piece)
Turmeric root, ½-inch (1 piece)
Coconut oil
Ingredients (raw):
Basil (1/2 bunch)
Coriander (1/4 bunch)
Peas, steamed (8 ounces)
Cucumber (1/2 piece)
Tomatoes (3 pieces)
Spinach, organic (1 handful)

Directions:
1. Add a bit of coconut oil to a skillet heated on medium. Stir in garlic and onions and cook for three minutes.
2. Stir in broccoli, carrots, cabbage, and cauliflower and cook for three minutes.
3. Pour in stock and tomatoes. Simmer for twenty minutes.
4. Process remaining ingredients in the blender until smooth. Add to the pot mixture and stir to combine.
5. Serve warm and topped with coriander.

Mock Sushi
Ingredients:
Rollups:
Avocado, peeled, sliced (1 piece)
Zucchini, medium, sliced thinly into long strips (2 pieces)

Carrot, julienned (1 piece)
Coriander/cilantro (1 bunch)
Capsicum, julienned (1 piece)
Cucumber, julienned (1 piece)
Hummus:
Peas, canned, drained (100 grams)
Cumin (1 pinch)
Almonds, raw (1 handful)
Olive oil (1 glug)
Garlic clove (1 piece)
Lemon juice (1 teaspoon)
Coconut aminos (1 tablespoon)
Himalayan sea salt (1 pinch)

Directions:
1. Place all hummus ingredients in the blender and process until smooth.
2. Lay zucchini strips on platter and smear with hummus.
3. Top with veggies, avocado, coriander, and sesame seeds.
4. Roll up and enjoy.

Hummus and Quinoa Wraps
Ingredients:
Quinoa, cooked (1 cup)
Hummus (1 cup) – *see* **Mock Sushi** *recipe above*
Avocado (1 cup)
Collard leaves, organic, large (4 pieces)
Sprouts, organic (1/2 cup)
Purple cabbage, organic, shredded (1/2 cup)
Beetroot, raw, finely sliced (1/2 cup)

Directions:
1. Spread hummus on top of collard leaves.
2. Add avocado, then quinoa, then all remaining ingredients to finish.
3. Roll to wrap and serve.

Quick Lettuce Salad
Ingredients:
Tomatoes, diced (2 pieces)
Avocado, diced (1 piece)
Lemon juice (1 ½ teaspoons)
Lettuces, little gem, organic, w/ leaves separated (2 pieces)
Radishes, chopped (2 pieces)
Cucumber, sliced (1/2 piece)
Carrot, julienned (1/2 piece)
Olive oil

Directions:
1. Place all ingredients in a salad bowl.
2. Gently toss to combine.
3. Serve and enjoy.

Lentil and Pumpkin Soup
Ingredients:
Soup:
Garlic cloves, minced (3 pieces + 1 piece)
Pumpkin seeds (1 teaspoon + 2 tablespoons)
Red onion, minced (1 piece)
Vegetable stock (300 milliliters)
Coconut cream (200 milliliters)

Pumpkin, chopped roughly (200 grams)
Carrots, chopped roughly (4 pieces)
Sweet potato, red, chopped roughly (1 piece)
Tomatoes, chopped roughly (4 pieces)
Bell pepper, red (1/2 piece)
Green peas, steamed (1 cup)
Coriander, fresh, chopped roughly (1 handful)
Turmeric root, fresh, 1-inch, chopped roughly (1 piece)
Ginger root, fresh, 1-inch, chopped roughly (1 piece)
Red chili, sliced thinly (1 piece)
Pine nuts, raw (1/2 cup)
Coconut oil

Directions:
1. Heat coconut oil in a skillet over medium heat. Stir in onion.
2. After thirty seconds, stir in garlic, ginger, turmeric, and pumpkin seeds. Cook for two minutes.
3. Stir in the sweet potato, carrot, pumpkin, and red pepper. Pour in stock and green peas after five minutes.
4. Simmer everything for fifteen minutes.
5. Stir in cilantro and coconut cream.
6. Serve and enjoy.

Scrumptious Springtime Soup
Ingredients:
Mint sprigs (2 pieces)
Peas, steamed (1 pound)
Avocado (1/2 piece)

Sea salt (1/4 teaspoon)
Black pepper (1/4 teaspoon)
Shallot (1 piece)
Cucumber (1/2 piece)
Olive oil (1 tablespoon)
Vegetable stock (250 milliliters)

Directions:
1. Fill blender with all ingredients.
2. Process until mixture is smooth.
3. Serve hot or cold.

Mint and Rocket Salad
Ingredients:
Rocket, organic (100 grams)
Olive oil (2 tablespoons)
Lemon juice, fresh (2 tablespoons)
Pepper, ground (1/4 teaspoon)
Himalayan sea salt (1/4 teaspoon)
Filtered/alkaline water (100 grams)
Peas, steamed (100 grams)
Mint, fresh (1/2 bunch)

Directions:
1. Add all ingredients to a salad bowl.
2. Gently toss to combine.
3. Serve right away.

Baby Peas and Quinoa Salad
Ingredients:
Avocado, diced (1 piece)
Baby peas, steamed (1 handful)

Black pepper (1 pinch)
Basil (1 handful)
Sage leaves (1 pinch)
Cherry tomatoes, grilled (15 pieces)
Quinoa, cooked (1 cup)
Carrot, spiralized (1 piece)
Beetroot, spiralized (1 piece)
Sea salt (1 pinch)
Dressing:
Olive oil (1 tablespoon)
Lemon juice (1 tablespoon)

Directions:
1. Fill a large bowl with lemon juice and olive oil. Mix well.
2. Add all remaining ingredients. Toss to combine.
3. Enjoy.

Raw Avocado Soup
Ingredients:
Lemon juice, freshly squeezed (2 teaspoons)
Celtic sea salt (1 pinch)
Pepper, freshly ground (1/4 teaspoon)
Avocados (3 pieces)
Tomatoes (3 pieces)
Spinach, organic, fresh (2 handfuls)
Filtered/alkaline water (as needed)

Directions:
1. Chop tomatoes into small chunks. Set aside.

2. Process remaining ingredients in the food processor. Pour into serving bowl.
3. Serve topped with tomato chunks.

Zucchini and Arugula Pasta
Ingredients:
Basil leaves (12 pieces)
Tomatoes, chopped (4 pieces)
Rocket leaves, organic (2 handfuls)
Garlic cloves (2 pieces)
Zucchini noodles (4 serves)
Courgette, chopped (1 piece)
Arugula, organic (1 bag)
Red onion, diced (1/2 piece)
Asparagus (1 bunch)
Olive oil

Directions:
1. Add courgette, asparagus, garlic, and basil in a blender filled with olive oil, pepper, and sea salt. Process until thick and smooth.
2. Pour on zucchini noodles and toss to combine.
3. Serve topped with rocket, red onion, and tomato.

Easy Lettuce Tacos
Ingredients:
Coconut aminos (4 tablespoons)
Lettuce leaves, organic (2 pieces)
Pine nuts, raw, chopped (3/4 cups)

Celery, chopped (1 ½ cups)
Onions, minced
Garlic, minced
Coconut oil
Ginger, chopped

Directions:
1. Pour a little alkaline/filtered water and coconut oil into a skillet heated on medium.
2. Stir in garlic, ginger, and onions. Cook for two minutes.
3. Add celery and cook for fifteen minutes.
4. Stir in pine nuts and cook for three minutes before adding coconut aminos.
5. Fill lettuce leaf with mixture and roll.

Pesto Zoodles
Ingredients:
Pine nuts/almonds, raw (1/4 cup)
Olive oil (1/4 cup)
Garlic clove, crushed (1 piece)
Sea salt (1 pinch)
Zucchinis, peeled, 6-inch, spiralized (2 pieces)
Celtic sea salt (1 pinch)
Basil leaves (1 cup)
Hemp hearts, raw (3 tablespoons)

Directions:
1. Add all ingredients except the spiralized zucchini to a food processor. Blitz until well-blended.

2. Pour pesto onto zucchini and toss to coat well.
3. Season to taste before serving.

Spinach Tofu Burgers
Ingredients:
Garlic cloves, minced (3 pieces)
Flaxseeds (1/8 cup)
Sunflower seeds (1/8 cup)
Paprika (1 tablespoon)
Sea salt (1/4 teaspoon)
Pepper (1/4 teaspoon)
Spinach, organic (16 ounces)
Tofu, firm, crumbled (15 ounces)
Millet (3/4 cup)
Onion, medium, chopped (1 piece)
Cumin (1 teaspoon)
Coconut oil (1/4 cup)
Coconut aminos (1/4 teaspoon)

Directions:
1. Toss all ingredients in a large bowl. Let sit for two minutes.
2. Shape mixture into patties.
3. Add a bit of coconut oil to a skillet heated on medium. Add patties and cook for ten minutes on each side.

Wow Wrapless Wraps
Ingredients:
Chili, fresh (1/2 piece)
Parsley, fresh, chopped (1/2 bunch)

Coriander, fresh, chopped (1/2 bunch)
Lemon juice (1 tablespoon)
Sea salt (1 pinch)
Romaine lettuce leaves, organic, large (6 pieces)
Tomatoes, ripe, chopped (2 pieces)
Avocados, ripe, mashed (3 pieces)
Red onion, medium, chopped (1/2 piece)

Directions:
1. Drizzle avocado with sea salt and lemon juice.
2. Add all chopped veggies and mix well.
3. Pat dry the lettuce leaves and fill with veggie mixture.
4. Wrap over and enjoy.

Indian Style Tofu Dish
Ingredients:
Spinach, organic, washed, roughly chopped (300 grams)
Tomatoes, skinned, cubed (2 pieces)
Coconut milk (100 milliliters)
Coriander (1 teaspoon)
Tofu, cubed (200 grams)
Onion, minced (1 piece)
Garlic clove, minced (1 piece)
Grapeseed oil (2 tablespoons)
Turmeric (1 teaspoon)
Chili powder (1/4 teaspoon)
Sea salt (1/4 teaspoon)
Black pepper (1/4 teaspoon)

Directions:
1. Pour oil into a wok heated on medium. Add tofu and cook until lightly golden. Drain on paper towels.
2. Add garlic, onion, and spinach to the same oil in the wok. Cook for one minute, then push tofu mixture to the wok's edges.
3. Add tomatoes and coconut milk to the wok's center. Simmer until thickened into a sauce, then stir in chili and other spices. Drag tofu mixture back to the wok's center and mix with the sauce.
4. Serve immediately.

Simply Awesome Sushi
Ingredients:
Capsicum, red, deseeded, sliced thinly into strips (1/2 piece)
Carrot, grated coarsely (1/3 cup)
Coconut aminos (3 tablespoons) – for serving
Brown rice, cooked (1 cup)
Nori sheets (4 pieces)
Avocado, ripe, peeled, mashed (1 piece)
Cucumber, sliced thinly into strips (1/2 piece)

Directions:
1. Toss avocado with the cooked brown rice.
2. Set nori sheets, matte side up, on a clean cutting board.
3. With wet hands, spread avocado rice on nori sheets. Top with capsicum, cucumber, and carrot.

4. Roll filled nori sheets and seal by brushing warm alkaline/filtered water on the edges. Let sit for five minutes.
5. Slice each roll into 6 pieces.
6. Enjoy by dipping in coconut aminos.

Warm Courgette and Red Pepper Salad
Ingredients:
Carrots, sliced (350 grams)
Olive oil, extra virgin (150 milliliters)
Himalayan sea salt (1/4 teaspoon)
Red pepper, w/ seeds removed (1 piece)
Courgettes, sliced into thick batons (450 grams)
Baby spinach, organic, fresh, washed, drained (300 grams)
Pepper, freshly ground (1/4 teaspoon)

Directions:
1. Line a serving dish (shallow) with spinach leaves.
2. Add olive oil to an oven-safe dish (wide) heated on low. Stir in peppers, carrots, pepper, and sea salt. Cover and cook for thirty minutes.
3. Stir in courgette pieces. Cover and cook for ten more minutes.
4. Serve immediately.

Fantastic Fennel and Brown Rice
Ingredients:
Olive oil (2 tablespoons)
Celtic sea salt (1/4 teaspoon)

Black pepper, freshly ground (1/4 teaspoon)
Fennel bulbs, large, quartered (6 pieces)
Onion, large, minced (1 piece)
Garlic cloves, minced (2 pieces)
Parsley, fresh, minced (1 bunch)
Brown rice, cooked
Vegetable stock, yeast-free

Directions:
1. Add olive oil to a frying pan heated on medium.
2. Stir in the onions and cook for two minutes.
3. Add garlic and fennel pieces; stir and cook for two minutes.
4. Pour in hot stock, cover, turn heat down to low, and cook for twenty minutes,
5. Stir in parsley, pepper, and sea salt.
6. Serve over cooked rice.

Perfect Pistou Soup
Ingredients:
Carrot, chopped finely (1 piece)
Onion, large, chopped finely (1 piece)
Celery stick, chopped finely (1 piece)
New potatoes, cubed (180 grams)
Broccoli sprouts, organic, chopped (450 grams)
Garlic cloves, crushed 3 pieces)
Olive oil, extra virgin (2 tablespoons)
Courgettes, cubed (200 grams)
Basil, fresh, chopped finely (1 bunch)
Sea salt (1/4 teaspoon)
Black pepper, freshly ground (1/4 teaspoon)

Vegetable stock, yeast-free (850 milliliters)
Tomatoes, large, skinned, deseeded, chopped (2 pieces)
Pistou:
Garlic cloves, large (2 pieces)
Olive oil, extra virgin (50 milliliters)
Basil leaves, fresh (100 grams)
Pine nuts, raw (1 ½ tablespoons)

Directions:
1. Process pistou ingredients in the blender until well-mixed. Transfer to individual bowls, cover with foil, and let sit in the refrigerator.
2. Add oil to a large pot heated on medium. Stir in garlic, celery, onion, and carrot. Cook for five to eight minutes.
3. Add stock, tomatoes, potatoes, pepper, and sea salt. Let mixture boil before adding the basil. Turn heat down to low, cover pot, and let soup simmer for ten minutes.
4. Stir in broccoli sprouts and courgette. Cook for ten minutes.
5. Season to taste and ladle into serving bowls. Top each with one tablespoon of pistou.

Spicy Peas and Aubergine Stew
Ingredients:
Olive oil (4 tablespoons)
Tomatoes, chopped (1200 grams)
Cumin, ground (1/2 teaspoon)

Coriander, ground (1/2 teaspoon)
Peas, soaked overnight, boiled, drained (200 grams)
Aubergines, large, cubed (3 pieces)
Onions, chopped (3 pieces)
Garlic cloves, chopped (2 pieces)
Cinnamon, ground (1/2 teaspoon)
Himalayan sea salt (1/4 teaspoon)
Black pepper, freshly ground (1/4 teaspoon)
<u>Garnish:</u>
Olive oil (2 tablespoons)
Coriander, fresh (3 sprigs)
Onion, sliced finely (1 piece)
Garlic clove, sliced finely (1 piece)
<u>For serving:</u>
Brown rice, cooked

Directions:
1. Place aubergine pieces in a colander and sprinkling with sea salt. Let stand for twenty minutes, then rinse and drain well.
2. Add oil to a large saucepan heated on medium. Stir in garlic and onion; cook for two minutes. Stir in all spices and aubergine cubes and cook for five minutes.
3. Stir in peas, tomatoes, pepper, and sea salt. Cover and simmer for twenty to twenty-five minutes.
4. Add all garnish ingredients in another skillet and cook over medium heat. Remove garlic and onion once golden.

5. Fill serving bowl with cooked brown rice. Pour in the stew and top with prepared garnish.

Chard and Chicory Veggie Platter
Ingredients:
Shallot, minced (1 piece)
Rucola leaves, organic, cut in two (60 grams)
Pepper, freshly ground (1/4 teaspoon)
Chicory leaves, organic, chopped (1 piece)
Chard leaves, organic (800 grams)
Pink grapefruit, w/ white skin removed & fruit filets cut out (700 grams)
Garlic clove, minced (1 piece)
Celtic sea salt (1/4 teaspoon)
Nutmeg, freshly ground (1/4 teaspoon)
Lemon peel, ground (1 tablespoon)
Lemon juice, freshly squeezed (1 tablespoon)

Directions:
1. Add olive oil to a skillet heated on medium.
2. Add garlic and shallot and cook for two minutes.
3. Stir in chard and cover for one minute.
4. Add spices and chicory and let simmer for two minutes.
5. Stir in remaining ingredients and cook for another five minutes.
6. Season to taste before serving.

Spring Greens with Brown Rice
Ingredients:
Onions, medium, sliced thinly (2 pieces)
Garlic cloves, chopped finely (2 pieces)
Red chili, fresh, seeded, sliced finely (1 piece)
Lemon juice, fresh (1 ½ tablespoons)
Celtic sea salt (1/4 teaspoon)
Spring green leaves, chopped finely (500 grams)
Grapeseed oil (2 tablespoons)
Water, alkaline/filtered (6 tablespoons) or vegetable stock, yeast-free (6 tablespoons)
Black pepper, freshly ground (1/4 teaspoon)
Brown rice, cooked

Directions:
1. Pour water/stock into a large saucepan heated on medium. Add the spring greens, cover, and cook for ten minutes.
2. In a separate saucepan, heat oil on medium. Stir in garlic, onion, and chili and cook for three to four minutes.
3. Stir in spring greens, cover, and cook for ten minutes.
4. Stir in black pepper, sea salt, and lemon juice.
5. Serve and enjoy.

Split Pea and Courgette Soup
Ingredients:
Vegetable stock, yeast-free (900 milliliters)
Turmeric, ground (1/2 teaspoon)
Himalayan sea salt (1/4 teaspoon)
Black pepper, freshly ground (1/4 teaspoon)

Onion, chopped finely (1 piece)
Courgettes, medium, diced finely (2 pieces)
Yellow split peas, soaked overnight, drained (1 cup)
Olive/rapeseed oil (1 tablespoon)

Directions:
1. Add oil to a large pot heated on medium. Add onion and cook for two minutes.
2. Set aside a handful of diced courgettes (boil and drain just before soup is finished). Toss the rest into the pot and cook for three minutes.
3. Pour in stock and turmeric. Let everything boil, then turn heat down to medium-low, cover, and simmer for thirty-five minutes.
4. Stir in black pepper, sea salt, and reserved courgettes. Cook for another one minute.
5. Serve right away.

Kale and Chickpea Rolls
Ingredients:
Rolls:
Vegetable stock, yeast-free (3/4 cup)
Brown rice (1/2 cup)
Paprika, ground (1/2 teaspoon)
Cumin, ground (1 teaspoon)
Onion, medium, chopped finely (1 piece)
Kale leaves, organic, large (12 pieces)
Peas, steamed (1 cup)
Olive oil, extra virgin (1 teaspoon)
Celtic sea salt (1/4 teaspoon)
Tomato salsa:

Plum tomatoes (1 can)
Jalapeno peppers (3 pieces)
Onion (1 piece)
Coriander (1 bunch)

Directions:
1. Add oil to a saucepan heated on medium. Stir in onion and cook for four minutes. Add stock, brown rice, peas, cumin, paprika, and sea salt. Let mixture boil, cover, and turn heat down to medium-low. Let everything simmer for fifteen minutes. Set aside to cool.
2. Process all tomato salsa ingredients in the blender.
3. Add rice mixture on top of each kale leaf. Fold, roll, set on a platter, and serve with tomato salsa.

Garlicky Spinach Salad
Ingredients:
Olive oil, extra virgin (4 tablespoons)
Celtic/Himalayan sea salt (1/4 teaspoon)
Black pepper, freshly ground (1/4 teaspoon)
Baby spinach leaves, organic, rinsed, drained (500 grams)
Garlic cloves, unpeeled (10 pieces)
Pine nuts, raw, toasted lightly (40 grams)
Lemon juice (1 tablespoon)

Directions:
1. Set oven at 350 degrees Fahrenheit to preheat.

2. Toss garlic and oil (2 tablespoons) in a roasting dish. Bake for ten to fifteen minutes.
3. Add roasted garlic to a salad bowl filled with spinach, pine nuts, lemon juice, olive oil, black pepper, and sea salt. Toss everything to combine.
4. Serve and enjoy.

Asparagus and Leeks Soup
Ingredients:
Vegetable stock, yeast-free (4 mugs)
Himalayan sea salt (1/4 teaspoon)
Pepper, freshly ground (1/4 teaspoon)
Green asparagus stalks and tips, fresh, chopped (800 grams)
Leeks, peeled, chopped (3 pieces)
Lemon (1/2 piece)
Olive oil (2 tablespoons)

Directions:
1. Add oil (2 tablespoons) to a large skillet heated on medium. Stir in leeks and cook for ten to fifteen minutes,
2. Pour in stock and asparagus pieces. Cover and simmer for twenty-five minutes.
3. Turn off heat and process soup with a hand blender. Season to taste.
4. Serve drizzled with lemon juice.
5. Enjoy.

Asparagus and Avocado Soup

Ingredients:
Baby spinach leaves, organic (1 handful)
Onions, dried (1/4 cup)
Garlic cloves (3 pieces)
Pepper, green/red (1 piece)
Green asparagus spears, medium (10 pieces)
Tomatoes (5 pieces)
Avocados, ripe (2 pieces)
Parsley/coriander, fresh (1 bunch)
Celtic/Himalayan sea salt (1/4 teaspoon)
Lemons, sliced thinly (2 pieces)
Mixed herbs, fresh

Directions:
1. Process all ingredients, except the lemon slices, in the food processor.
2. Pour mixture into a pot and heat on medium-low.
3. Serve soup garnished with lemon slices.

Creamy Lettuce Salad with Almonds
Ingredients:
Lemon juice (1 tablespoon)
Olive oil, cold-pressed (4 tablespoons)
Celtic sea salt (1/4 teaspoon)
Black pepper, freshly ground (1/4 teaspoon)
Lamb's lettuce, organic, chopped (600 grams)
Almonds, raw, chopped (200 grams)
Parsley/chives, fresh, chopped (1 bunch)
Avocados, cubed (2 pieces)

Directions:
1. Combine lemon juice, fresh herbs, sea salt, pepper, and olive oil to make the dressing.
2. Toss remaining ingredients in a salad bowl.
3. Add dressing to the salad and mix well.
4. Serve right away.

Spicy Spelt Pasta Salad
Ingredients:
Baby spinach, organic (1 handful)
Red onion, medium, chopped (1 piece)
Garlic cloves, minced (2 pieces)
Chili, small, sliced (1 piece)
Spelt/vegetable pasta, cooked (200 grams)
Aubergine, large, cubed (1 piece)
Red pepper, sliced (1 piece)
Tomatoes, cubed (3 pieces)
Vegetable stock, yeast-free (150 milliliters)
Basil leaves, fresh, torn (1 handful)
Sea salt (1/2 teaspoon)
Coconut oil (1 teaspoon)
Cayenne pepper (1 pinch)
Olive oil, extra virgin (1 drizzle)

Directions:
1. Add coconut oil to a pan heated on medium. Stir in garlic, onion, and aubergine and cook for two minutes.
2. Stir in stock, tomato, capsicum, cayenne pepper, and sea salt.
3. Let everything simmer for twelve minutes.

4. Add the spinach and basil and cook for one minute. Pour over cooked pasta.
5. Serve dish drizzled with olive oil.

Stir-Fried Buckwheat Noodles
Ingredients:
Olive/flaxseed oil (1 tablespoon)
Coconut aminos (1 tablespoon)
Sea salt (1/4 teaspoon)
Pepper (1/4 teaspoon)
Olive oil (1 tablespoon)
Mixed veggies (carrots, fennel, bean sprouts, and courgette), organic, chopped
Garlic, chopped finely (2 pieces)
Onions, chopped finely (2 pieces)
<u>Buckwheat noodles:</u>
Buckwheat flour (100 grams)
Water, filtered/alkaline (50 milliliters)

Directions:
1. Fill a large bowl with buckwheat flour. Make a well in the middle and fill with water. Mix well and knead into a pliable dough. Cover with cling film before refrigerating for thirty minutes.
2. Roll out dough on a clean surface dusted with a little buckwheat flour. Once evenly thick, cut dough into long, thin strips.
3. Set a bowl of cold water in the sink.
4. Heat a small pot filled with alkaline/filtered water on medium-high. Once boiling, add the buckwheat noodles and reduce heat to medium. Once cooked,

transfer the noodles into the bowl of cold water.
5. Add olive oil to a frying pan heated on medium. Stir in garlic and onions and cook for thirty seconds.
6. Stir in carrots and cook for another thirty seconds.
7. Add remaining veggies and stir-fry for thirty seconds before adding the drained buckwheat noodles.
8. Season dish with sea salt, pepper, and coconut aminos before serving.

Pesto Courgette Rolls
Ingredients:
Courgettes, large, cut into long & thin strips (1 piece)
Pesto filling:
Olive oil, cold-pressed (50 milliliters)
Himalayan sea salt (1 pinch)
Pine nuts, raw (70 grams)
Garlic cloves (3 pieces)
Basil, fresh (1/4 cup)
Parsley, fresh (1/4 cup)
Red pepper dip:
Lemon juice, freshly squeezed (3 teaspoons)
Celtic sea salt (1/4 teaspoon)
Black pepper, freshly ground (1/4 teaspoon)
Garlic clove, minced (1 piece)
Red pepper, small (1 piece)

Directions:
1. Process all pesto filling ingredients in the food processor until creamy.
2. Smear courgette strips with pesto filling on one side. Roll and secure with toothpicks before setting on a platter.
3. Blend all red pepper dip ingredients in the food processor. Serve with the rolls.
4. Enjoy.

Alfalfa and Cress Salad
Ingredients:
A mixture of cress and alfalfa, organic
Lemon juice (1 tablespoon)
Celtic sea salt (1/4 teaspoon)
Black pepper, freshly ground (1/4 teaspoon)
Cucumber (1 piece)
Spring onion (1 piece)
Chives, fresh (1 teaspoon)
Dill, fresh (1 teaspoon)
Parsley, fresh (1 teaspoon)
Coconut oil (2 tablespoons)

Directions:
1. Mince all herbs before mixing with the lemon juice, oil, pepper, and sea salt.
2. Slice cucumber and spring onion into small bits, then stir into the dressing.
3. Place all remaining ingredients in a salad bowl. Toss with the dressing.

Green Kohlrabi Salad
Ingredients:
Sprouts, organic, fresh (4 tablespoons)
Himalayan sea salt (1/4 teaspoon)
Olive oil (3 tablespoons)
Green kohlrabi, organic (3 pieces)
Shallot/spring onion (1 piece)
Lemon juice, fresh (1 tablespoon)
Black pepper, freshly ground (1/4 teaspoon)

Directions:
1. Slice the peeled kohlrabi into thin pieces.
2. Mince the shallot/spring onion. Mix with all remaining ingredients.
3. Serve kohlrabi with dressing and enjoy.

Artichoke and Radicchio Salad
Ingredients:
Jerusalem artichokes, cut roughly to same size (500 grams)
Lemon juice (1 tablespoon + 1 tablespoon)
Lemon rind, grated (1 tablespoon)
Sea salt (1/4 teaspoon + ¼ teaspoon)
Black pepper, freshly ground (1/4 teaspoon)
Radicchio leaves, organic (150 grams)
Coconut oil (3 tablespoons)
Parsley, flat-leaf – for serving

Directions:
1. Preheat the grill on high.
2. Line a flame-proof dish with the radicchio leaves. Scatter almonds on top before

sprinkling with oil, pepper, and sea salt. Grill for three minutes.
3. Fill a pot with alkaline/filtered water. Add sea salt (1/4 teaspoon) and lemon juice (1 tablespoon). Heat to boiling, then add the artichokes to cook for five to seven minutes.
4. Add artichokes, lemon zest, and lemon juice (1 tablespoon) to the salad. Season to taste before grilling until browned.
5. Serve and enjoy.

Moroccan Spiced Courgettes
Ingredients:
Courgettes (500 grams)
Parsley, fresh, chopped (1 handful)
Coriander, fresh, chopped (1 handful)
Lemon juice, freshly squeezed (2 tablespoons)
Dressing:
Paprika (1/2 teaspoon)
Cumin, ground (1/2 teaspoon)
Olive oil (3 tablespoons)
Onion (1 piece)
Garlic cloves, minced (2 pieces)
Red/green chili, seeded, sliced finely (1/4 piece)
Himalayan sea salt (1/4 teaspoon)
Black pepper, ground (1/4 teaspoon)

Directions:
1. Set oven at 350 degrees Fahrenheit to preheat.
2. Slice courgettes into lengthwise quarters before adding to a shallow dish.

3. Mince the onion and mix with alkaline/filtered water and other ingredients for the dressing.
4. Smother courgettes with the dressing. Cover and cook in the oven for fifteen minutes.
5. Use dressing to baste the courgette dish. Bake, uncovered, for five to ten minutes.
6. Serve topped with chopped herbs and drizzled with lemon juice.

Collar Apple Wrap

Ingredients:
Sea salt (1/8 teaspoon)
Sweet onion, sliced thinly (1 piece)
Almonds, raw (1 cup)
Apple, medium, sliced thinly (2 pieces)
Coconut vinegar (1/8 teaspoon)
Collard greens, organic (4 leaves)

Directions:
1. Slice each leaf in half and discard the stem.
2. Stuff remaining ingredients into the leaves.
3. Serve wraps right away.

Minty Wheat Berry Salad

Ingredients:
Stevia (1 tablespoon)
Mint, fresh, chopped finely (1/2 cup)
Sea salt (1/2 teaspoon)

Water, alkaline/filtered (3 cups)
Blueberries (1 cup)
Olive oil (2 tablespoons)
Celery, diced (1 cup)
Ginger root, minced (2 teaspoons)
Green onion/ramp/scallion, chopped finely (1/2 cup)
Apple, chopped finely (2 cups)
Apple juice (2 tablespoons)

Directions:
1. Add blueberries to a ceramic bowl and cover with alkaline/filtered water (2 inches). Refrigerate overnight.
2. Drain blueberries and add to a saucepan. Pour in alkaline/filtered water (3 cups) and sea salt/ Heat to boiling, then turn heat down to low. Simmer for forty-five minutes.
3. Drain the blueberries and place in a large bowl. Stir in the apples, green onion, celery, and mint.
4. Whisk together the remaining ingredients, then pour on top of the salad.
5. Refrigerate for four hours before serving.

Chapter 4 Alkaline Diet-Aligned Dinner Recipes

Warm Cherry Tomatoes and Broccoli Salad

Ingredients:
Lemon juice, fresh (2 tablespoons)
Parsley, fresh, chopped (2 tablespoons)
Oregano, dried (1 teaspoon)
Thyme, dried (1 teaspoon)
Broccoli florets, organic, fresh, steamed briefly (400 grams)
Onion, cubed (1 piece)
Cherry tomatoes, chopped (100 grams)
Olive oil, cold-pressed (1 tablespoon)
Himalayan sea salt (1/4 teaspoon)

Directions:
1. Add the crunchy steamed broccoli florets to a salad bowl.
2. Pour in a mixture of herbs, lemon juice, sea salt, pepper, and olive oil.
3. Gently toss to blend everything.
4. Serve and enjoy.

Veggie Primavera

Ingredients:
Coconut/olive oil (1/2 tablespoon)
Garlic clove, minced (1 piece)
Asparagus, trimmed, cubed (1 bunch)
Carrots, large, peeled, julienned (3 pieces)

Leeks, medium, rinsed, sliced thinly into rounds (1 piece)
Green peas, steamed (1 cup)
Sea salt
Pepper, ground
Pesto:
Olive oil, extra virgin (2 tablespoons)
Hemp seeds, hulled (1/4 cup)
Basil, fresh (3/4 cup)
Garlic clove (1 piece)
Water, alkaline/filtered (1 tablespoon)
Lemon juice, fresh (1 tablespoon)
Sea salt (1/4 teaspoon)
Sundried tomato, oil-packed, drained (1/4 cup)

Directions:
1. Add oil to a skillet heated on medium. Stir in garlic and leek and cook for three to four minutes.
2. Stir in asparagus, sea salt, and pepper. Turn heat up to medium-high; after eight minutes of cooking, add the green peas.
3. Combine the pesto ingredients in the food processor.
4. Place carrot pasta on a platter and serve topped with pesto.

Zoodles Stuffed Tomatoes

Ingredients:
Marinated zucchini:
Oregano, minced (1 tablespoon)
Dill, minced (1 tablespoon)

Zucchini, fresh, sliced into half-moon shapes (2 pieces)
Yellow squash, fresh (2 pieces)
Tomatoes, sundried, chopped (1/2 cup)
Olive oil (1 tablespoon)
Basil, minced (1 tablespoon)
Sea salt (1 teaspoon)
Nutty cheese:
Lemon juice, freshly squeezed (1/4 cup)
Bell pepper, red, chopped (1/2 piece)
Sea salt (1 teaspoon)
Water, filtered (1/3 cup)
Pine nuts, raw (1 cup)
Tomato cups:
Dill (1/4 teaspoon)
Black pepper (1/4 teaspoon)
Paprika (1/4 teaspoon)
Tomato, medium (1 piece)

Directions:
1. Process all nutty cheese ingredients in the blender. Set aside.
2. Toss zucchini with the sundried tomatoes and spices. Let sit for one hour.
3. Slice tomato in half. Scoop out the flesh (reserve the skins for your tomato cups) and chop along with the marinated zucchini. Combine with nutty cheese.
4. Fill the tomato cups with the filling. Serve garnished with dill, black pepper, and paprika.

Polenta with Asparagus and Mushroom Sauce

Ingredients:
Asparagus:
Asparagus, trimmed, chopped (1 bunch)
Olive oil (1 tablespoon)
Mixed herbs (1 pinch)
Garlic powder (1 dash)
Onion powder (1/8 teaspoon)
Mushrooms:
Cremini mushrooms (227 grams)
Olive oil (1 tablespoon)
Mixed herbs (1 pinch)
Parsley, dried (1/4 teaspoon)
Vegetable stock (1/4 cup)
Apple cider vinegar (2 tablespoons)
Polenta:
Vegetable stock (1 ½ cups)
Olive oil (1 tablespoon)
Brown rice flour (1 cup)
Sea salt (1 teaspoon)
To serve:
Micro-greens, organic
Herbs

Directions:
1. Coat asparagus with olive oil, garlic powder, onion powder, and mixed herbs. Spread on greased baking pan and bake at 375 degrees Fahrenheit for thirty-five to forty minutes, stirring halfway.
2. Add oil to a skillet heated on medium. Stir in mushrooms and cook for two minutes. Stir in seasonings, apple cider vinegar,

and veggie broth. Simmer for five minutes.
3. Fill a saucepan with olive oil, sea salt, and vegetable stock. Heat to boiling, then gradually whisk in the brown rice flour. Keep whisking until the polenta mixture is creamy.
4. Pour polenta onto your serving dish and top with asparagus. Serve drenched in mushroom sauce and garnished with herbs/micro-greens.
5. Enjoy.

Ancho Chili Chard Wrap
Ingredients:
Wrap:
Red pepper, small, sliced thinly (1/2 piece)
Chard leaves, organic, large (2 pieces)
Avocado (1/2 piece)
Cucumber, 4-inch, sliced into 10 slender strips (1 piece)
Radish & sunflower sprouts, organic
Dip:
Ancho chili powder (3/4 teaspoon)
Olive oil (2 tablespoons)
Alkaline water (2 tablespoons)
Almond butter, raw (3 tablespoons)
Ginger, raw, grated (3/4 teaspoon)
Garlic, raw, grated (3/4 teaspoon)
Stevia (3 drops)
Lemon juice, fresh (1 tablespoon)

Directions:

1. Mix all dip ingredients in a bowl. Set aside.
2. Line a large plate with chard leaves. Fill with veggies and roll to form wraps. Secure with toothpicks.
3. Serve wraps with dip and enjoy.

Amazing Aubergine Pizza
Ingredients:
Pepper, green/red (1 piece)
Red onion (1 piece)
Black olives (1 handful)
Aubergine, large (1 piece)
Tomatoes (2 pieces)
Garlic cloves (2 pieces)
Basil (1 handful)
Rocket, organic (2 handfuls)
Tomato puree/paste, homemade
Coconut oil
Alkaline/filtered water

Directions:
1. Set oven at 350 degrees Fahrenheit to preheat.
2. Slice aubergine to form 2/3-cm pieces, brush lightly with oil, spread on baking sheet, and bake for fifteen to twenty minutes.
3. Fill a small saucepan with coconut oil (1 tablespoon), alkaline/filtered water (1 tablespoon), tomatoes, pepper, red onion, garlic, and half of basil. Stir and cook for two minutes.

4. Top aubergine pieces with the sautéed veggies. Bake for five minutes.
5. Top with rocket and basil. Serve sprinkled with olive oil, pepper, and sea salt.

Sham Sushi
Ingredients:
Nori sheets (8 pieces)
Green cabbage head, organic, medium (1/2 piece)
Cucumber (1 piece)
Tamari, wheat-free (3 tablespoons)
Chili (1 teaspoon)
Bean sprouts, organic (1 cup)
Avocado (1 piece)
Lemon juice (1 tablespoon)
Cilantro (1/2 cup)
Filling:
Carrots, medium (1 piece)
Sesame seeds (2 tablespoons)
Almonds, raw (3 cups)
Garlic powder (1 teaspoon)
Ginger root, 1-cm, sliced (1 piece)
Parsley, fresh, minced (3 tablespoons)
White onion, medium, chopped (1/2 piece)
Lemon juice (3 tablespoons)
Olive oil (3 tablespoons)
Tamari, wheat-free (2 tablespoons)
Dill, fresh, chopped (2 tablespoons)
Basil, fresh, chopped (2 tablespoons)
Directions:
1. Set aside onion, sesame seeds, and herbs.

2. Place the rest of the filling ingredients in a food processor. Blitz until well-blended, then add to a large bowl. Stir in the reserved ingredients and let sit in the fridge for five days.
3. Lay out nori sheets on a cutting board. Top each with a cabbage leaf, then smear with filling mixture. Add cucumber slices, chili, tamari, lemon juice, avocado slices, sprouts, and cilantro. Roll and slice into sushi-like pieces.
4. Serve and enjoy.

Cherry Sea Veggies Salad
Ingredients:
Salad:
Green onion, sliced (1 piece)
Watercress, organic, chopped (1 cup)
Black sesame seeds (1 teaspoon)
White sesame seeds (1 teaspoon)
Dried seaweed, soaked, drained (15 milliliters)
Wakame seaweed, raw, soaked, drained (15 milliliters)
Beets, raw, julienned (3 pieces)
Radish, medium, julienned (1 piece)
Dressing:
Coconut aminos (1/2 cup)
Apple cider vinegar (1/4 cup)
Stevia (3 teaspoons)
Lemon juice (2 tablespoons)
Ginger root, chopped (1/4 cup)
Sour cherry, dried (1/2 cup)
Stevia (3 teaspoons)

Garlic clove (1 piece)
Sesame oil (1/4 cup)
Cherry marinade:
Sour cherry, dried (1/2 cup)
Stevia (4 teaspoons)
Apple cider vinegar (1/4 cup)

Directions:
1. Fill a bowl with cherry marinade ingredients. Let sit for one hour and drain.
2. Process all dressing ingredients in the blender.
3. Add the remaining ingredients, except the sesame seeds, in a large bowl. Add the cherry marinade and toss to combine.
4. Serve garnished with sesame seeds.

Delish Pesto Sweet Potato Casserole
Ingredients:
Himalayan sea salt (¼ teaspoon)
Green peas, steamed (15 ounces)
White onion, medium, diced (1 piece)
Sweet potato, cubed (3 cups)
Coconut milk (1/4 cup)
Pumpkin seeds (1 cup)
Garlic cloves, peeled, chopped (2 pieces)
Himalayan sea salt (1/2 teaspoon)
Pesto:
Garlic cloves, peeled, chopped (3 pieces)
Olive oil (1/2 cup)
Lemon juice (3 tablespoons)
Pine nuts, raw (1/2 cup)

Basil, fresh (2 cups)
Himalayan sea salt (1/2 teaspoon)

Directions:
1. Process pesto ingredients in the blender.
2. Set oven at 350 degrees Fahrenheit to preheat.
3. Fill a large saucepan with a little alkaline/filtered water. Add garlic and sweet potatoes, making sure they are just covered with water. Heat to boiling, then turn heat down to a simmer. Cover and cook for twenty minutes.
4. Process coconut milk, pesto (1/2 cup), and pumpkin seeds in the blender. Set aside.
5. Add coconut oil to a frying pan heated on medium. Stir in onion and cook for two minutes. Stir in green peas and sea salt and cook for five minutes. Spread mixture onto a baking tray. Top with pesto mixture.
6. Bake for twenty minutes.
7. Serve and enjoy.

Broccoli Sprouts Salad
Ingredients:
Parsley, chopped (1/2 bunch)
Broccoli sprouts, organic (2 cups)
Baby arugula, organic (2 cups)
Asparagus, thin, w/ ends trimmed (1 bunch)
Olive oil (1/4 cup)
Lemon zest (1 tablespoon)
Lemon juice, fresh (2 tablespoons)

Sea salt (1/4 teaspoon)
Black pepper (1/4 teaspoon)

Directions:
1. Fill a pot with alkaline/filtered water and heat to boiling. Add asparagus and cook for five to eight minutes.
2. Pat dry asparagus before chopping into one-inch chunks.
3. Whisk together parsley, olive oil, and lemon.
4. Place asparagus, arugula, and broccoli sprouts in a large bowl. Add the dressing and gently toss to combine.
5. Season to taste and serve.

Lime and Chipotle Cauliflower
Ingredients:
Cauliflower:
Avocado oil (2 tablespoons)
Cauliflower, large (1 piece)
Seasoning:
Garlic powder (1/4 teaspoon)
Chipotle powder (1/2 tablespoon)
Himalayan salt (1/4 teaspoon)
Garnish:
Lime, freshly squeezed (2 tablespoons)

Directions:
1. Set oven at 325 degrees to preheat.
2. Line baking sheet with parchment.
3. Combine all seasoning ingredients.

4. Chop cauliflower into one-inch chunks and place in a bowl. Toss with avocado oil and seasoning mixture, then spread out on cookie sheet.
5. Bake for one hour and thirty minutes.
6. Serve drizzled with lime juice.

Appetizing Broccoli Soup
Ingredients:
Onion, chopped (1 piece)
Sweet potato, peeled, cubed (1 piece)
Thyme, dried (1 teaspoon)
Vegetable broth, yeast-free (4 cups)
Broccoli florets, organic (4 cups)
Green peas, steamed (15 ounces)
Garlic cloves, minced (3 pieces)
Celery seeds, whole (1 teaspoon)
Sea salt (1 ½ teaspoons)
Turmeric powder (1/4 teaspoon)
Oregano (1/2 teaspoon)
Black pepper, ground (1/4 teaspoon)

Directions:
1. Fill a large pot with vegetable broth, green peas, sweet potato, garlic, onion, black pepper, turmeric, thyme, marjoram, and celery seeds. Heat on medium, cover, and cook for twenty minutes. Let sit to slightly cool.
2. Process soup in the blender until smooth. Pour back into the pot and heat on medium. Stir in green peas and sea salt,

then cover and cook for five to ten minutes.
3. Serve right away.

Pineapple and Asian Kale Slaw
Ingredients:
Pineapple, diced (1 cup)
Broccoli sprouts, organic, steamed (1 cup)
Sesame seeds, toasted (1 tablespoon)
Kale, sliced thinly (2 cups)
Carrots, medium, shredded (2 pieces)
Napa cabbage, organic, raw, shredded (1 cup)
Dressing:
Ginger root, minced (1 teaspoon)
Almond butter (1 ½ tablespoons)
Stevia (1 tablespoons)
Lime juice (2 tablespoons)
Tamari, wheat-free (1 tablespoon)
Rice vinegar (3 tablespoons)
Olive oil (2 tablespoons)
Sesame oil (2 teaspoons)
Lime zest (2 tablespoons)

Directions:
1. Process all dressing ingredients in the blender.
2. Mix together the carrots, cabbage, kale, pineapple, broccoli sprouts, and sesame seeds in a large bowl. Add dressing and toss until well-coated.
3. Let sit on the counter for ten minutes, then serve.

Nutty Lemon and Apple Salad
Ingredients:
Pumpkin seeds, chopped (1/3 cup)
Almonds, raw, chopped (1/3 cup)
Olive oil (2 tablespoons)
Lemon juice, fresh (2 tablespoons)
Green apple, large, chopped (2 pieces)
Cucumber, chopped (3 pieces)
Yellow bell pepper, medium, sliced (1 piece)
Sesame seeds (1/3 cup)
Chives, chopped finely (1 tablespoon)
Sea salt (1/2 teaspoon)
Rosemary, fresh, chopped (1 tablespoon)

Directions:
1. Cube the bell pepper, apples, and cucumbers.
2. Roughly chop up the almonds, pumpkin seeds, and sesame seeds.
3. Stir the sea salt, olive oil, chives, lemon juice, and rosemary together in a large bowl. Add the chopped veggies, nuts, and seeds. Toss to combine.

Avocado and Papaya Salad with Arugula
Ingredients:
Lime juice, fresh (3 tablespoons)
Papaya, ripe, medium, divided (4 pieces)
Shallots, small, chopped (2 pieces)
Yellow onion, medium, chopped finely (1 piece)
Arugula, organic, chopped coarsely (1 cup)
Avocado, small, diced (2 pieces)

Pine nuts, raw, chopped (1/3 cup)
Cilantro, fresh, chopped coarsely (1/4 cup)

Directions:
1. Slice 2 papayas in half and remove seeds. Set aside.
2. Peel the other 2 papayas. Slice in half and remove seeds as well. Chop into half-inch cubes and add to a bowl filled with pine nuts, shallots, cilantro, lime juice, and avocados. Gently toss to combine and season to taste before folding in the arugula.
3. Stuff salad in the reserved unpeeled papaya halves.

Beet Kale and Red Kuri Salad
Ingredients:
Cranberries (1 ½ cups)
Garlic, minced (1 teaspoon)
Green apples, medium, sliced thinly (1 piece)
Kale, organic, w/ stems removed, chopped roughly (8 cups)
Apple cider vinegar (1/4 cup)
Beets, raw, peeled, cubed (4 pieces)
Cinnamon (2 teaspoons)
Coconut sugar (1/4 cup)
Lemon juice, fresh (1 ½ tablespoons + 1 ½ tablespoons + 1 cup)
Nutmeg, ground (1/4 teaspoon)
Pumpkin seeds (3 cups)
Kuri squash, red, seeded, cubed (1 piece)
Rosemary, dried (1 teaspoon)

Coconut yogurt (1 cup)
Cooking spray, olive oil (2 sprays)
Orange juice, fresh (1 cup)
Sea salt (1/8 teaspoon)
Pepper (1/8 teaspoon)

Directions:
1. Set oven at 400 degrees Fahrenheit to preheat.
2. Use parchment paper to line 2 baking sheets.
3. Spread the beet cubes on one sheet and the red kuri squash pieces on the other sheet. Drizzle both with olive oil. Sprinkle rosemary on top of the beets and nutmeg and cinnamon of the squash. After seasoning with pepper and sea salt, bake for thirty minutes, stirring halfway. Let cool within ten minutes.
4. Add kale to a large bowl and toss with olive oil (1 teaspoon) and lemon juice. Let stand for ten minutes.
5. Fill a small saucepan with coconut sugar and orange juice; stir to combine. Heat to boiling, then add cranberries and simmer for five to seven minutes. Set aside to cool.
6. Process all remaining ingredients in the food processor until crumbly. Add to the kale bowl.
7. Add veggies and apple slices to the kale bowl as well. Toss to combine everything and serve right away.

Potatoes and Peas Stew

Ingredients:

Yellow/red pepper, w/ seeds & stalk removed, sliced into rings (1 piece)
Courgette, cubed (1 piece)
Red chili, fresh, small, sliced finely (1 piece)
Sesame oil (3 tablespoons)
Onions, large, sliced into rings (3 pieces)
New potatoes, medium, cubed (2 pieces)
Peas, steamed (200 grams)
Carrots, large, cubed (1 piece)
Black pepper, ground (1 pinch)
Cumin, ground (1 pinch)
Cardamom, ground (1 pinch)
Sea salt (1 tablespoon)
Coriander, ground (1 pinch)
Ginger, ground (1 pinch)

Directions:

1. Add sesame oil to a skillet heated on medium. Stir in onions and cook for two minutes.
2. Stir in sea salt, peppercorns, chili, cardamom, cumin, coriander, and ginger and cook for two minutes.
3. Stir in courgette, potato, carrot, and pepper and cook for two minutes. Add alkaline/filtered water (1 cup) for deglazing.
4. Stir in peas and more alkaline/filtered water (1 cup). Cook for another five minutes.
5. Serve and enjoy.

Asian Style Mushrooms
Ingredients:
Ginger, fresh, diced (50 grams)
Lemongrass stalks, sliced thinly (2 pieces)
Lime peel, fresh (from 4 limes)
Coconut aminos (2 tablespoons)
Mushrooms, chopped (800 grams)
Coriander, fresh, chopped finely (30 grams)
Red chilis, deseeded, sliced finely (2 pieces)
Black peppercorns, crushed (1 teaspoon)
Sea salt (20 grams)
Oyster sauce (1 tablespoon)
Sesame seeds, toasted (1 handful)
Olive oil (2 tablespoons)
Garlic, minced (2 cloves)
Onion, minced (1/4 cup)

Directions:
1. Combine coriander, coconut aminos, lime peel, lemongrass, chili, ginger, pepper, and sea salt.
2. Place mushrooms in a bowl. Add marinade and let sit in the fridge for two days.
3. Drain marinated mushrooms and sprinkle with sesame seeds.
4. Add oil to a skillet heated on medium. Stir in onion and garlic and cook for two minutes. Add mushrooms and stir-fry for five minutes.
5. Serve and enjoy.

Green Peas Ratatouille
Ingredients:
Brown rice (1 mug)
Water, alkaline (1 mug)
Olive oil (2 tablespoons)
Rosemary, chopped (1 handful)
Red peppers, cubed (2 pieces)
Leek, sliced into thin rings (1 piece)
Green peas (15 ounces)
Tomatoes, chopped (15 ounces)
Ginger, ground (1 pinch)
Black pepper, freshly ground (1/4 teaspoon)
Cinnamon (1 pinch)
Sea salt (1/4 teaspoon)

Directions:
1. Follow package directions in cooking brown rice.
2. Cook leeks and peppers in olive oil over medium heat. Stir in tomatoes and cook on a simmer for five minutes.
3. Stir in green peas and simmer for another five to ten minutes.
4. Remove from heat and stir in pepper, sea salt, ginger, cinnamon, and rosemary.
5. Serve and enjoy.

Mouthwatering Sweet Potato Soup
Ingredients:
Olive oil (2 tablespoons)
Sweet potatoes, peeled, cubed (400 grams)
Vegetable stock, yeast-free, hot (200 milliliters)
Coconut cream (200 milliliters)

Garlic cloves (2 pieces)
Onion, sliced (1 piece)
Ginger, ground (2 pinches)
Chili flakes, dried (2 pinches)
Black pepper, freshly ground (1/4 teaspoon)
Spinach leaves, organic (30 grams)
Coriander leaves, fresh, chopped (50 grams)
Himalayan sea salt (1/4 teaspoon)

Directions:
1. Add oil to a saucepan on medium heat. Stir in onion and garlic and cook for three to four minutes.
2. Stir in ginger and chili flakes and cook for one minute.
3. Stir in sweet potato and cook for two to three minutes.
4. Pour in coconut milk and stock. Let everything boil, reduce heat, and simmer for eight to ten minutes.
5. Stir in coriander and turn off heat. Process with a hand blender and season to taste.
6. Serve garnished with spinach.

Green Peas Curry Stew
Ingredients:
Ginger, fresh, grated (1/2 teaspoon)
Cumin, ground (1/2 teaspoon)
Chili, fresh (1/2 teaspoon)
Turmeric powder (1/2 teaspoon)
Carrot, big, finely grated (1 piece)
Red onion, sliced finely (1 piece)

Leek, sliced into thin rings (1 piece)
Garlic cloves, sliced finely (2 pieces)
Curry powder (1 teaspoon)
Olive oil, extra virgin (2 tablespoons)
Black pepper, freshly ground (1/4 teaspoon)
Himalayan sea salt (1/4 teaspoon)
Green peas (250 grams)
Water, filtered/alkaline (1 1/5 liters)

Directions:
1. Add olive oil to a large pot heated on medium. Stir in onions and cook for four to five minutes. Add leek, garlic, and carrot and cook for two minutes. Stir in chili, cumin, turmeric, curry powder, ginger, and alkaline/filtered water and cook for two minutes.
2. Stir in green peas and let mixture boil. Reduce heat to a simmer, cover, and cook for thirty-five minutes.
3. Let stew slightly cool before processing with a hand blender. Cook for another two minutes to heat through and season to taste.
4. Serve and enjoy.

Delicious Fennel Soup
Ingredients:
Orange juice, fresh (2 tablespoons)
Orange peel, ground finely (1 teaspoon)
Fennel bulbs, shredded (2 pieces)
Vegetable stock, yeast-free (2/8 liter)
Lemon juice, fresh (4 tablespoons)

Flax seed oil (1/2 teaspoon)
Coriander, ground
Pepper

Directions:
1. Add vegetable stock to a pot heated on medium. Stir in lemon juice and let mixture boil.
2. Add fennel and cook for ten to fifteen minutes.
3. Process mixture with a hand blender.
4. Stir in flax seed oil, orange juice, pepper, and coriander.
5. Serve garnished with orange peel.

Curried Romanesco Cauliflower
Ingredients:
Peas, steamed (3 handfuls)
Parsley, chopped (1 handful)
Curry powder (1/2 tablespoon)
Garam masala (1/2 tablespoon)
Romanesco cauliflower, medium, chopped into florets (1 piece)
Garlic cloves, sliced finely (2 pieces)
White/red onion, chopped (1 piece)
Ginger, fresh, minced (1 tablespoon)
Lemon peel, grated (1 teaspoon)
Black pepper, freshly ground (1/4 teaspoon)
Olive/rapeseed oil (1 tablespoon)
Chili, fresh, sliced finely (1 piece)
Celtic sea salt (1/4 teaspoon)

Directions:
1. Set oven at 390 degrees Fahrenheit to preheat.
2. Fill a large bowl with cauliflower, garlic, ginger, onions, curry powder, pepper, garam masala, sea salt, oil, lemon peel, and chili. Toss to combine and spread on a baking tray.
3. Roast for twenty-five minutes, stirring halfway. Stir in peas.
4. Serve topped with coriander and enjoy.

Comforting Pumpkin Soup
Ingredients:
Red chilis, deseeded, sliced finely (2 pieces)
Garlic cloves, minced (3 pieces)
Brown rice (1 mug)
Olive oil (4 tablespoons)
Pumpkin, deseeded, cubed (1 kilogram)
Onion, large, finely chopped (1 piece)
Carrots, sliced (4 pieces)
New potatoes, cubed (4 pieces)
Vegetable stock, yeast-free (1 ¼ liters)
Celtic sea salt (1 pinch)
Parsley, chopped finely (1 handful)

Directions:
1. Add olive oil to a skillet heated on medium.
2. Stir in garlic and onion and cook for two minutes.
3. Stir in rice, pumpkins, potatoes, carrots, and chilis and cook for ten minutes.

4. Pour in stock, pepper, and sea salt. Reduce heat to low and continue cooking for thirty minutes.
5. Stir in parsley and turn off heat. Let sit for five minutes before serving.

Ginger Greens Stir-Fry
Ingredients:
Cabbage, organic (1/4 piece)
Mixed leafy greens, organic (2 handfuls)
Red/green chili, minced (1 piece)
Coconut oil (2 tablespoons)
Squash, deseeded, chopped into 1-cm pieces (1/2 piece)
Onion, minced (1 piece)
Ginger, 2-cm, peeled, chopped (1 piece)
Garlic cloves, peeled, chopped (3 pieces)
Lemon juice (1 tablespoon)
Sea salt (1/4 teaspoon)
Pepper, freshly ground (1/4 teaspoon)
Alkaline/filtered water (1 liter)
Coconut aminos (1 dash)

Directions:
1. Add coconut oil to a large skillet heated on medium-low. Stir in onion and cook for two minutes. Add garlic, ginger, and chili and cook for one minute.
2. Stir in sea salt (1 pinch) and squash. Cook for five minutes.
3. Add leafy greens and a little lemon juice and gently toss to combine. Season with coconut aminos, pepper, and sea salt.

4. Stir in mixed leafy greens and cook for one minute.
5. Serve right away.

Tasty Tunisian Chickpea Soup
Ingredients:
Carrots, sliced finely into strips (2 pieces)
Celery stalks, sliced thinly into rings (5 pieces)
Onions, chopped finely (2 pieces)
Chard/kale stalks, organic, sliced roughly (2 pieces)
Peas, steamed (350 grams)
Garlic cloves, sliced finely (10 pieces)
Olive oil (8 tablespoons)
Cumin, ground (1 teaspoon)
Turmeric (1/2 teaspoon)
Lemon juice (1 tablespoon)
Sea salt, Himalayan/Celtic (1/4 teaspoon)
Black pepper, freshly ground (1/4 teaspoon)
Coriander, ground (1 teaspoon)
Coriander, chopped finely (4 tablespoons)

Directions:
1. Add half of olive oil to a large pot heated on medium. Stir in garlic and cook for two minutes. Stir in peas, coriander, cumin, turmeric, and alkaline/filtered water. Let mixture boil, then reduce heat to a simmer and continue cooking for two hours and thirty minutes.
2. Add remaining oil to a skillet heated on medium. Stir in onions, celery,

chard/kale, and carrots and cook for five minutes.
3. Add veggie mixture to soup mixture and cook for ten minutes. Process with a hand blender, then stir in lemon juice, pepper, and sea salt.
4. Serve topped with fresh coriander.

Broccoli and Mushrooms Dish
Ingredients:
Broccoli, organic, chopped into florets, steamed (500 grams)
Parsley, fresh (1 handful)
Chives, fresh (1 handful)
Mushrooms (400 gramso
Olive oil (2 tablespoons)
Grapeseed/rapeseed oil (2 tablespoons)
Lemon slices (2 pieces)
Lemon juice (2 tablespoons)
Black pepper, freshly ground (1/4 teaspoon)
Celtic/Himalayan sea salt (1/4 teaspoon)

Directions:
1. Combine olive oil and lemon juice. Add mushrooms and let sit for twenty minutes.
2. Add grapeseed/rapeseed oil to a frying pan heated on low. Drain mushrooms and stir into pan to cook for five to eight minutes. Add mushroom marinade and let mixture cook for two minutes. Season to taste and place on a serving plate filled with steamed broccoli.

3. Serve smothered with sauce from the pan and garnished with lemon slices, parsley, and chives.

Almond and Broccoli Spelt Pasta
Ingredients:
Almonds, raw, flaked (150 grams)
Garlic cloves, minced (2 pieces)
Avocado (2 tablespoons)
Broccoli florets, organic, chopped (800 grams)
Spelt pasta, cooked (250 grams)
Sea salt (1/4 teaspoon)
Black pepper, freshly ground (1/4 teaspoon)

Directions:
1. Add avocado oil to a skillet heated on medium-low. Stir in garlic and cook for one minute. Add broccoli and a little alkaline/filtered water; stir and cook for five minutes.
2. Add almonds to a separate skillet heated on medium; cook until roasted.
3. Toss broccoli mixture with the cooked spelt pasta. Season to taste and top with almonds.
4. Serve and enjoy.

Curried Root Vegetable with Brown Rice
Ingredients:
Red chili, chopped roughly (1 piece)
Onion, large, minced (1 piece)
Tomatoes, chopped (15 ounces)

Coriander, fresh (1 bunch)
Mixed root veggies, diced (7 handfuls)
Grapeseed/rapeseed oil (3 tablespoons)
Garlic cloves, large, chopped (3 pieces)
Cinnamon sticks (2 pieces)
Turmeric, ground (3 teaspoons)
Cumin seeds (2 teaspoons)
Coconut milk (15 ounces)
Lime (1 piece)
Sea salt (1/4 teaspoon)
Pepper, freshly ground (1/4 teaspoon)
Fennel seeds (1 teaspoon)
Coriander (2 teaspoons)
Ginger, fresh, chopped (1 piece)
Brown rice, cooked

Directions:
1. Set oven at 390 degrees Fahrenheit to preheat. Place a roasting tray inside.
2. Place diced root veggies in a large bowl. Toss with oil, pepper, and sea salt. Add to preheated tray and shake well. Roast for forty minutes.
3. Add fennel seeds, cumin, and coriander to a frying pan heated on medium. Stir and cook for two minutes, grind to a coarse powder, and stir in the turmeric.
4. Process onion, garlic, ginger, and chili in the blender until pureed.
5. Add a little oil to a skillet heated on medium-low. Stir in spices and cook for one minute. Stir in spicy paste and cook for five minutes.

6. Add tomatoes, coconut milk, and cinnamon to the pan and cook for two minutes, stirring constantly. Season to taste before pouring all over roasted veggies.
7. Bake dish for twenty-five minutes.
8. Serve sprinkled with lime juice and coriander leaves.

Coconut Curry Carrots
Ingredients:
Garlic cloves, minced (3 pieces)
Coconut milk, unsweetened (200 milliliters)
Vegetable stock, yeast-free (200 milliliters)
Lemon zest (1/2 teaspoon)
Lemon juice, fresh (1 tablespoon)
Broccoli florets, organic (500 grams)
Carrots, sliced thinly (400 grams)
Onions, medium, sliced (2 pieces)
Sea salt (1/4 teaspoon)
Black pepper, freshly ground (1/4 teaspoon)
Coconut oil (2 tablespoons)
Curry powder (2 tablespoons)

Directions:
1. Add oil (2 tablespoons) to a skillet heated on medium. Stir in garlic, onion, and curry powder to cook for two minutes.
2. Stir in carrots, broccoli, and a little sea salt. Cook for five minutes, then add stock, coconut milk, and lemon zest. Cover and cook for twelve minutes.

3. Stir in pepper, sea salt, curry powder, and lemon juice. Cook until boiling, then remove from heat.
4. Serve immediately.

Sweet Potato Curry and Coconut Quinoa
Ingredients:
Garlic cloves, minced (2 pieces)
Coconut oil (2 tablespoons)
Coriander (1 teaspoon)
Cumin (1 teaspoon)
Peas, steamed (15 ounces)
Quinoa, dry (1/2 cup)
Sweet potato, medium, steamed, cubed (1 piece)
Onion, medium, chopped (1/2 piece)
Turmeric (1 teaspoon)
Garlic powder (3/4 teaspoon)
Cayenne (1/2 teaspoon)
Sea salt (1/4 teaspoon)
Pepper, freshly ground (1/4 teaspoon)
Cardamom (1/8 teaspoon)
Ginger (1/8 teaspoon)
Coconut milk (15 ounces)

Directions:
1. Add alkaline/filtered water (300 milliliters) to a saucepan heated on medium-high. Add quinoa, sweet potatoes, and peas and cook until boiling. Cover, reduce heat to a simmer, and cook for fifteen minutes.
2. Add coconut oil to a skillet heated on medium. Stir in garlic and onion and cook

for two minutes. Add all spices and cook for two minutes.
3. Add quinoa mixture to the pan, then pour in coconut milk. Stir to combine and cook until boiling. Reduce heat to low, cover, and cook for ten to fifteen minutes.
4. Serve and enjoy.

Broccoli with Coconut Scented Rice
Ingredients:
Broccoli heads, organic, chopped, steamed (3 pieces)
Carrot, medium, grated (4 pieces)
Sesame seeds (1 teaspoon)
Lime slices – to squeeze and for garnish
Sauce:
Water, filtered/alkaline (150 milliliters)
Lemon juice (50 milliliters)
Coriander, ground (1 ½ teaspoons)
Cumin (3/4 teaspoon)
Coconut aminos (125 milliliters)
Olive oil (40 milliliters)
Chili pepper (1/3 teaspoon)
Coconut scented rice:
Almonds, raw, finely chopped, lightly toasted (1/4 cup)
Mint, fresh, finely chopped (3 sprigs)
Brown rice, rinsed (1 cup)
Coconut milk (2 cups)
Shredded coconut (1/4 cup)

Directions:
1. Set oven at 350 degrees Fahrenheit to preheat.
2. Place carrots and broccoli in a large bowl.
3. Process all sauce ingredients in the food process until thick and creamy. Stir in sesame seeds and set aside.
4. Add sauce to the veggie bowl and toss to combine. Top with lime slices and sprinkle with lime juice.
5. Mix together coconut scented rice ingredients, except for the almonds, in a saucepan and heat on high. Let mixture boil, cover, and reduce heat to a simmer. Cook for twenty-five minutes. Use a fork to fluff rice before sprinkling with almonds and mint.
6. Serve broccoli with coconut scented rice.

Alkaline Diet-Friendly Quinoa Stew
Ingredients:
Tomatoes, fresh, chopped (2 pieces)
Cabbage, sliced finely (1/4 piece)
Broccoli head, organic, shaved (1/2 piece)
Garlic cloves, crushed, chopped (2 pieces)
Coconut oil (1 teaspoon)
Brown onion, minced (1 piece)
Celery stalk, chopped (1 piece)
Carrots, chopped (2 pieces)
Quinoa, uncooked (1/2 cup)
Water, alkaline/filtered (750 milliliters)
Tomatoes, tinned, chopped (15 ounces)
Green peas, drained (15 ounces)

Cumin, ground (1 teaspoon)
Sea salt (1/4 teaspoon)
Black pepper (1/4 teaspoon)
Avocado (1/2 piece)
Olive oil (1 drizzle)
Sunflower seeds (1 teaspoon)
Cilantro, fresh, chopped roughly (1 bunch)

Directions:
1. Fill a large soup pot with coconut oil and heat on medium. Stir in onion, garlic, celery, and carrots and cook for three to four minutes. Add cumin and sunflower seeds and cook for two to three minutes.
2. Stir in fresh tomatoes, green peas, cabbage, and quinoa. Cook for two minutes, then add tinned tomatoes and alkaline/filtered water. Season with pepper and sea salt and let everything simmer for ten minutes.
3. Stir in broccoli and 2/3 of cilantro. Pour into individual bowls and top with avocado.
4. Serve sprinkled with oil and cilantro.

Alfredo Zucchini Noodles
Ingredients:
Garlic cloves, minced (3 pieces)
Pine nuts, raw, soaked overnight, rinsed (1/4 cup)
Almond milk (2 ½ cups)
Vegetable stock cube, yeast-free (1 piece)
Cauliflower, organic, medium, chopped (1 piece)

Avocado oil (1 tablespoon)
Coconut oil (1 tablespoon)
Oregano, fresh (1 tablespoon)
Basil, fresh (1 tablespoon)
Himalayan sea salt (1/4 teaspoon)
Black pepper (1/4 teaspoon)
Lemon juice (2 tablespoons)
Zucchini noodles – to serve

Directions:
1. Add oil to a pot heated on medium. Stir in garlic and cook for two to three minutes. Stir in almond milk and stock cube. Let mixture simmer.
2. Add pine nuts and cook for six to eight minutes.
3. Process all remaining ingredients in the blender until smooth.
4. Serve on top of zucchini noodles.

Broccoli Pumpkin Soup
Ingredients:
Broccoli florets, organic (4 cups)
Pumpkin, chopped (3 cups)
Vegetable broth, gluten-free (4 cups)
Almond milk (2 cups)
Coconut oil (1 tablespoon)
Onion, medium, chopped (1 piece)
Garlic cloves, minced (2 pieces)
Celery, chopped (1 cup)
Cayenne pepper flakes (1/4 teaspoon)
Lemon juice (1/2 tablespoon)
Pink sea salt (1/4 teaspoon)

Black pepper (1/4 teaspoon)
Parsley, fresh, chopped (1/4 cup + 1 teaspoon)

Directions:
1. Add oil to a large pot heated on medium. Stir in onion and cook for five to six minutes. Add garlic to cook for one minute, then stir in pumpkin, celery, parsley (1/4 cup), coconut yogurt, cayenne, and broth. Cook for ten to twelve minutes.
2. Add broccoli to the soup and cook for five minutes. Process with a hand blender.
3. Stir in almond milk. Cook for another two minutes or until heated through.
4. Stir in sea salt, black pepper, and lemon juice.
5. Serve topped with chopped parsley (1 teaspoon).

Succulent Spaghetti Squash Patties
Ingredients:
Coriander, fresh (3 grams)
Flax seed, ground (1 teaspoon)
Leeks, finely chopped (30 grams)
Spaghetti squash (1 piece)
Za'atar (1/4 teaspoon)
Spring onion, sliced thinly (1 piece)
Ginger, grated (4 grams)
Coriander (1 teaspoon)
Sunflower oil (2 tablespoons)
Dressing:
Lemon juice (1 piece)

Himalayan sea salt (1 pinch)
Coconut aminos (3 tablespoons)
Water, alkaline/filtered (5 tablespoons)

Directions:
1. Set oven at 350 degrees Fahrenheit to preheat.
2. Slice spaghetti squash into halves and remove the seeds. Sprinkle sunflower oil (1 tablespoon) on top and bake for forty minutes. Let cool before scooping out flesh with a fork to form spaghetti strands.
3. Add leeks, spring onion, coriander, ginger, zatar, and flax seed to the squash. Refrigerate for a while.
4. Whisk all dressing ingredients together.
5. Add remaining sunflower oil to a pan heated on medium. Shape squash mixture into patties and add to the pan and cook for two minutes on each side.
6. Serve and enjoy.

Spinach and Soba Noodle Dish
Ingredients:
Spring onions, sliced thinly (4 pieces)
Cucumber, julienned (1/2 piece)
Carrot, spiralized (1 piece)
Broccoli, organic, chopped (1/2 piece)
Red cabbage, organic, sliced thinly (1/4 piece)
Spinach leaves, organic (2 handfuls)
Tomatoes, sliced (2 pieces)
Red onion, diced (1/2 piece)

Broccoli sprouts, organic (1 handful)
Coriander leaves (1 handful)
Lime juice (2 tablespoons)
Coconut aminos (3 tablespoons)
Alfalfa sprouts, organic (1 handful)
Buckwheat noodles, cooked – to serve

Directions:
1. Tear coriander leaves and toss with lime juice. Let sit for five minutes.
2. Place remaining ingredients in a salad bowl. Add the buckwheat noodles and marinated coriander and gently toss to combine.
3. Serve and enjoy.

Yummy Sweet Potato Pasta
Ingredients:
Tomatoes, sundried, halved, softened in warm alkaline/filtered water, chopped (7 pieces)
Lemon juice (1 teaspoon)
Olive oil (1 teaspoon + 1 teaspoon)
Oregano (1/2 teaspoon)
Sweet potato, spiralized (1 piece)
Roma tomatoes, chopped (2 pieces)
Almonds, raw (1/4 cup)
Basil (1/2 teaspoon)
Sea salt (1/2 teaspoon)
Red pepper flakes (1 dash)
Water, alkaline/filtered

Directions:

1. Process almonds in the blender until flour-like. Add olive oil (1 teaspoon), seasonings, and lemon juice and process until well-combined.
2. Add chopped sundried tomatoes and Roma tomatoes to the blender and process until creamy.
3. Pour sauce on top of sweet potato noodles. Serve sprinkled with remaining olive oil and red pepper flakes.

"Cheesy" Rotini Mushroom Casserole
Ingredients:
Casserole:
Spelt pasta (16 ounces)
Mushrooms, sliced (8 ounces)
Onion, medium, peeled, quartered (1 piece)
Garlic cloves, large (3 pieces)
Basil, dried (1/2 teaspoon)
Oregano, dried (1/2 teaspoon)
Broccoli, organic (1 cup)
Paprika (1/4 teaspoon)
White pepper (1/4 teaspoon)
Sea salt (1/4 teaspoon)
Breadcrumbs, gluten-free: (1/4 cup)
Almond flour (1/8 cup)
Cayenne pepper, ground (1/8 teaspoon)
Himalayan pink salt (1/4 teaspoon)
Nutritional yeast (1/8 cup)
Garlic powder (1/4 teaspoon)
"Cheesy sauce":
Almond milk (2 cups)
Garlic clove, large (1 piece)

Smoked paprika (1 teaspoon)
Coconut yogurt (1/3 cup)
Pine nuts, raw (1/4 cup)
Cornstarch (1 tablespoon)
Coconut aminos (5 teaspoons)

Directions:
1. Set oven at 350 degrees Fahrenheit to preheat.
2. Mix all breadcrumbs ingredients and set aside.
3. Fill a large pot with alkaline/filtered water and heat to boiling. Stir in a little sea salt. Add spelt pasta and cook for six minutes.
4. Process broccoli, onions, garlic, and mushrooms in the blender until coarsely ground. Pour into a sauté pan heated on medium and filled with a little alkaline/filtered water and cook for seven to ten minutes.
5. Process "cheesy sauce" ingredients in the blender.
6. Drain cooked spelt pasta and pour into pan. Toss to coat with prepared sauce. Add to a casserole pan and top with prepared breadcrumbs. Sprinkle with smoked paprika and bake for twenty to twenty-five minutes.
7. Serve immediately.

Easy Spinach Pie
Ingredients:
Green peas, steamed, mashed (15 ounces)

Spinach (20 ounces)
Coconut yogurt (2 tablespoons)
Kalamata olives, chopped (1/3 cup)
Onion, minced (1 cup)
Green onions, diced (1 cup)
Garlic cloves, chopped (4 pieces)
Coconut aminos (1/3 cup)
Lemon juice (1/4 cup)
Black pepper (1/4 teaspoon)
Oregano, fresh, minced (2 tablespoons)
Parsley, fresh, minced (2 tablespoons)
<u>Flaxseed mixture:</u>
Stevia (2 tablespoons)
Flax seed meal (2 tablespoons)
Lemon juice (4 tablespoons)
<u>Pie crusts</u> (2 pieces):
Ground flax (4 tablespoons) + filtered water (5 tablespoons)
Salt (1 tablespoon)
Almond flour, fine (2 ½ cups)
Tapioca flour (2/3 cup)

Directions:
1. To prepare pie crust: Mix ground flax and water; let stand for five to ten minutes. Whisk together tapioca flour, almond flour, and salt. Stir in thickened flax and mix into a dough. Shape into two balls. Roll out each dough ball until wide enough to line a pie tin.
2. Press each rolled out dough onto pie tin and freeze for twenty minutes.
3. Set oven at 400 degrees Fahrenheit to preheat.

4. Cover each dough with foil; top with pie weights and bake for fifteen minutes. Set aside to cool.
5. Set oven at 350 degrees Fahrenheit to preheat.
6. Mist cooking spray onto a baking pan (9x9-inch).
7. Mix flaxseed meal, lemon juice, and stevia. Let stand for ten minutes to thicken.
8. Add alkaline/filtered water (2 tablespoons) to a skillet heated on medium. Stir in onion, garlic, and green onion and cook for five minutes. Stir in spinach to cook for another five minutes. Stir in spinach and other remaining ingredients, save for the dough, and cook for five minutes. Turn off heat and let slightly cool.
9. Line baking dish with one of the pie crusts. Brush a little flaxseed mixture on the surface before spreading on the spinach mixture. Top with the other pie crust and brush with flaxseed mixture.
10. Bake for thirty to forty minutes. Slice into squares and enjoy.

Mock Beef Stew

Ingredients:
Apple cider vinegar (2 tablespoons)
Almond flour (1/4 cup)
Vegetable broth, gluten-free (4 cups)
Olive oil (2 tablespoons)

Yellow onion, large, minced (1 piece)
Garlic cloves, minced (5 pieces)
Tomato paste (2 tablespoons)
Carrots, large, cubed (2 pieces)
Potatoes, cubed (3 ½ cups)
Black pepper (1 teaspoon)
Thyme (1 teaspoon)
Parsley, chopped (1/4 cup)
Celery stalks, cubed (3 pieces)
Bay leaves (3 pieces)
Tofu, firm (15 ounces)

Directions:
1. Add oil to a large pot heated on medium. Stir in onions and cook for five minutes.
2. Stir in tomato paste and garlic and cook for two minutes.
3. Add apple cider vinegar. Stir in almond flour and cook for one minute.
4. Stir in potatoes, carrots, bay leaves, thyme, celery, black pepper, and broth. Cook on a simmer, stirring frequently, for forty minutes.
5. Stir in tofu and parsley and cook for two more minutes.
6. Serve immediately.

Potato Cakes with Green Peas Stuffing
Ingredients:
Potato cakes:
Sea salt (1/4 teaspoon)
Potato starch (1 cup)
Potatoes, medium (10 pieces)

Bay leaf (1 piece)
<u>Stuffing:</u>
Olive oil (2 tablespoons)
Green peas, steamed (3/4 cup)
Salt (1/4 teaspoon)
Black pepper (1/4 teaspoon)
Onion, medium, chopped (1 piece)
Mushrooms (4 ounces)
Coconut oil

Directions:
1. Pour alkaline/filtered water (7 cups) into a large pot. Add potatoes, sea salt, and bay leaf. Heat to boiling; once potatoes are tender, remove from heat and rinse with cold water to easily remove skins.
2. Mash boiled potatoes. Mix with potato starch and stir into a dough.
3. Add olive oil to a sauté pan heated on medium-high. Stir in onion and cook for five minutes. Add mushrooms to cook for five minutes, then add green peas, pepper, and sea salt to cook for another two minutes. Let stuffing cool.
4. Press dough (3 tablespoons) into your palm. Add stuffing (1 tablespoon), fold over, and mold into a disk. Repeat with remaining dough and stuffing.
5. Add coconut oil to a skillet heated on medium. Add potato cakes and cook for four minutes on each side.

Thai Green Curried Veggies
Ingredients:
Broccoli head, organic (1 piece)
Zucchini, medium (1 piece)
Red bell pepper (1 piece)
Coconut milk (2 cups)
Vegetable stock, yeast-free (2 cups)
Green curry paste (3 teaspoons)
Sweet potato, small (1 piece)
Eggplant, small (1 piece)
Kaffir lime leaves, organic (3 pieces)
Ginger, fresh, 1-inch, grated (1 piece)
Sea salt (1/4 teaspoon)
Pepper, ground (1/4 teaspoon0
Lime juice (2 tablespoons)
Coconut aminos (3 tablespoons)
Brown rice, cooked – to serve

Directions:
1. Fill a large pot with vegetable stock and heat to boiling. Stir in kaffir lime leaves, ginger, coconut milk, and all chopped veggies. Cover, reduce heat to a simmer, and cook for twenty to thirty minutes.
2. Season pot mixture with pepper and sea salt. Cover and simmer for an additional five to ten minutes.
3. Remove from heat and stir in coconut aminos and lime juice.
4. Serve with cooked brown rice and enjoy.

Pesto Lemon Mushrooms
Ingredients:

Lemon zest, grated (1 tablespoon)
Garlic cloves, chopped roughly (2 pieces)
Olive oil (3 tablespoons)
Sea salt (1 pinch)
Portobello mushrooms, quartered (8 ounces)
Parsley, chopped roughly (1 ¼ cups)
Lemon juice (2 tablespoons)
Pine nuts, raw (1/2 cup)
Stevia (3 drops)

Directions:
1. Set oven at 350 degrees Fahrenheit to preheat.
2. Drain mushrooms and spread at the bottom of an oven-proof dish to form an even layer.
3. Process all remaining ingredients in the blender until well-combined and thick.
4. Spread pesto over mushroom surface. Bake for ten to fifteen minutes.
5. Serve and enjoy.

Luscious Layered Veggie Bake
Ingredients:
Beet, diced (1 piece)
Tamari, wheat-free (1/2 teaspoon)
Chives, dried (1 teaspoon)
Cumin, ground (1 pinch)
Green peas, steamed (1/2 cup)
Olive oil (4 tablespoons + 2 tablespoons)
Beefsteak tomato, chopped roughly (1 piece)
Garlic clove, chopped (1 piece)
Filtered/alkaline water (2 tablespoons)

Butternut squash, sliced thinly into lengthwise pieces (13 ounces)
Zucchini, sliced thinly into lengthwise pieces (10 ounces)

Directions:
1. Set oven at 350 degrees Fahrenheit to preheat.
2. Add green peas to a small pan. Add enough alkaline/filtered water to cover green peas and heat to boiling. Reduce heat to a simmer and cook for ten to fifteen minutes. Set aside after draining.
3. Add olive oil to a skillet heated on medium. Stir in tomato, beets, garlic, cumin, chives, and tamari. Add alkaline/filtered water and cook for fifteen minutes.
4. Stir in green peas and cook on a simmer for five minutes.
5. Add 1/3 of zucchini and ½ of butternut squash to a pie tin. Top with sauce. Repeat layering until all squash, zucchini, and sauce are used up.
6. Brush olive oil on top of dish and bake for forty-five minutes.
7. Serve and enjoy.

Veggie Fest Pizza
Ingredients:
Crust:
Almond meal (1/2 cup)
Cauliflower florets, organic (1 pound)

Chia/flax seeds, ground, divided (3 tablespoons)
Alkaline/filtered water (6 tablespoons)
Sea salt (1/2 teaspoon)
Garlic powder (1/2 teaspoon)
Oregano, dried (1/2 teaspoon)
Toppings:
Garlic cloves, sliced (2 pieces)
Oregano, dried (1 teaspoon)
Sea salt, fine (1 teaspoon)
Black pepper, ground (1/2 teaspoon)
Mushrooms, small, sliced (4 ounces)
Cherry tomatoes, halved (8 ounces)
Red onion, small, sliced into half-circles (1 piece)
Olive oil (1 tablespoon)
Basil leaves, fresh (1 cup)
Hot pepper flakes (1/4 teaspoon)
Lemon wedges (3 pieces)

Directions:
1. Set oven at 400 degrees Fahrenheit to preheat.
2. Use parchment paper to line your baking sheet.
3. Add cauliflower to a blender and process until rice-like. Pour into a large pot and cover with just enough alkaline/filtered water. Heat to boiling, cover, turn heat down to a simmer, and cook for five minutes. Drain the cauliflower and freeze for ten minutes.
4. Combine chia/flax seeds (2 tablespoons) and alkaline/filtered water (6 tablespoons). Let stand to thicken into an egg-like consistency.

5. Remove cauliflower from the freezer and squeeze out any excess moisture. Mix with chia/flax seed mixture and other crust ingredients. Spread onto a pie tin to form an even layer. Bake for fifteen to twenty minutes. Let crust cool.
6. Set oven at 350 degrees Fahrenheit to preheat.
7. Mix all topping ingredients together and spread onto a pie tin to form an even layer. Roast for thirty minutes, stirring halfway. Let slightly cool.
8. Set topping on top of crust and bake for another five minutes.

Easy Kale Salad
Ingredients:
Smoked paprika (1/2 teaspoon)
Garlic cloves (2 pieces)
Water, filtered (1 ¼ cups)
Brown rice syrup (1 ½ teaspoons)
Kale leaves, organic, torn (1 bunch)
Sunflower seeds (1 cup)
Almond nuts, raw (1/3 cup)
Red pepper flakes (1/4 teaspoon)
Sea salt (1/2 teaspoon)
To serve:
Sunflower seeds (1 teaspoon)

Directions:
1. Place torn kale leaves in a large bowl.
2. Process all remaining ingredients in the blender until smooth and creamy.

3. Top kale with dressing and toss to coat.
4. Let stand for ten minutes.
5. Serve sprinkled with sunflower seeds.

Spinach with Lemon and Peas
Ingredients:
Grape tomatoes (2 cups)
Lemon zest, grated (1 tablespoon)
Lemon juice, fresh (2 tablespoons)
Red pepper flakes, crushed (1 teaspoon)
Peas, steamed (15 ounces)
Olive oil (3 tablespoons)
Onion, large, sliced thinly (1 piece)
Garlic cloves, minced (4 pieces)
Ginger, grated (1 tablespoon)
Sea salt (1/4 teaspoon)

Directions:
1. Add olive oil to a skillet heated on medium. Stir in onion to cook for five minutes.
2. Stir in garlic, tomatoes, ginger, red pepper flakes, and lemon zest. Cook for three to four minutes.
3. Stir in peas and cook for three to four minutes.
4. Add spinach; once starting to wilt, stir in sea salt and lemon juice. Cook for two more minutes.
5. Serve immediately.

Spaghetti Squash Stuffed with Quinoa

Ingredients:

Green peas, steamed (1 cup)
Shallot, medium (1 piece)
Spaghetti squash, large, halved, deseeded (1 piece)
Coconut oil (2 tablespoons)
Quinoa, cooked (1 ½ cups)
Thyme, dried (2 teaspoons)
Garlic powder (1 teaspoon)
Pink sea salt (1/4 teaspoon)
Black pepper (1/4 teaspoon)
Red/orange bell pepper (1 piece)
Spring onions, white portion only, sliced (2 pieces)
Almonds, raw, chopped (1/4 cup)

Directions:

1. Set oven at 400 degrees Fahrenheit to preheat.
2. Place squash in roasting tin and bake for forty minutes.
3. Add oil (1 tablespoon) to a skillet heated on medium. Stir in bell pepper and shallot and cook for two minutes. Stir in green peas, quinoa, almonds, pepper, sea salt, and spices.
4. Top squash halves with the veggie mixture. Return to the oven and bake for five to eight minutes.
5. Serve and enjoy.

Courgette Pad Thai
Ingredients:
Cauliflower florets, organic (1 cup)
Coriander, chopped roughly (1 bunch)
Courgettes, medium, spiralized (3 pieces)
Carrots, large, spiralized (3 pieces)
Spring onions, chopped (2 pieces)
Red cabbage, organic, shredded (1 cup)
Coconut oil
Sauce:
Coconut sugar (1 teaspoon)
Lime/lemon juice (2 tablespoons)
Garlic clove, minced (1 piece)
Coconut aminos (1/4 cup)
Almond butter (1/4 cup)
Tamari, wheat-free (1/4 cup)
Ginger root, 1-inch, grated (1 piece)

Directions:
1. Add spiralized zucchini and carrots to a large bowl. Add the shredded cabbage, coriander, cauliflower, and spring onions as well.
2. Mix together the almond butter, coconut aminos, tamari, grated ginger, garlic, coconut sugar, and lime/lemon juice.
3. Add prepared sauce to the vegetable bowl. Toss to combine everything.
4. Serve and enjoy with a little lime/lemon juice.

Hearty Minestrone Dream
Ingredients:

Red onion (1/4 piece)
Garlic cloves (2 pieces)
Broccoli sprouts, organic (1/2 cup)
Coconut oil (1 tablespoon)
Eggplant (1/2 cup)
Sweet potato (1/2 cup)
Zucchini (1/2 cup)
Carrot (1/2 cup)
Vegetable stock, yeast-free (1 cup)
Basil (1 handful)
Tomato juice, fresh (1 cup)
Black pepper (1/4 teaspoon)
Himalayan sea salt (1/4 teaspoon)

Directions:
1. Cut the potato, courgette, and aubergine into cubes.
2. Dice the onion and carrot.
3. Add coconut oil to a large pot heated on medium. Stir in chopped veggies and cook for two minutes.
4. Stir in broccoli sprouts, tomato juice, and stock. Let mixture boil, then reduce heat to a simmer. Cook for another eight to ten minutes.
5. Stir in basil, pepper, and sea salt before serving.

Pesto Buckwheat Noodles and Pine Nuts Galore
Ingredients:
Olive oil (1 cup)
Basil (1 bunch)

Parsley (1 tablespoon)
Coriander (1 tablespoon)
Buckwheat noodles, cooked (1 serve)
Pine nuts, raw (250 grams)
Himalayan sea salt (1/4 teaspoon)
Pepper, freshly ground (1/4 teaspoon)

Directions:
1. Set buckwheat noodles on serving plate.
2. Process the remaining ingredients in the food processor until smooth and creamy.
3. Toss the noodles and pesto together until well-combined.
4. Serve and enjoy.

Ginger Pumpkin Soup
Ingredients:
Red chili, fresh, deseeded, sliced (1 piece)
Ginger, fresh, 1-cm, chopped roughly (1 piece)
Vegetable stock, yeast-free (1 2/5 liters)
Orange juice, fresh (2 tablespoons)
Butternut squash, medium, cubed (1 piece)
Carrots, large, cubed (2 pieces)
Red onion, large, minced (1 piece)
Garlic cloves, minced (3 pieces)
Thyme leaves, fresh (1 tablespoon)
Sea salt (1/4 teaspoon)
Pepper, freshly ground (1/4 teaspoon)
Coconut/olive oil

Directions:
1. Pour oil to a large pot and heat on medium.

2. Add onion and garlic and cook for two minutes. Stir in squash, carrot, sea salt, and pepper and cook for five minutes.
3. Pour in vegetable stock, chili, thyme, and ginger. Let mixture boil, then simmer for twenty-five minutes.
4. Process mixture with a hand blender before drizzling with orange juice.
5. Serve and enjoy.

Tantalizing Tuscan Bean Soup
Ingredients:
Carrot, chopped (1 piece)
Tomatoes, chopped (3 cups)
Broccoli sprouts, organic (6 cups)
Water, alkaline/filtered (5 cups)
Olive oil (2 tablespoons)
Onion, medium, chopped (1 piece)
Celery stalks, chopped (2 pieces)
Garlic cloves, chopped (4 pieces)
Himalayan sea salt (1/2 teaspoon)
Pepper, freshly ground (1/4 teaspoon)
Quinoa (1/2 cup)
Basil leaves, fresh, coarsely chopped (1/4 cup)

Directions:
1. Add onions, garlic, celery, and a splash of filtered/alkaline water to a skillet heated on medium. Steam-fry for two minutes.
2. Stir in carrots and tomatoes and cook for fifteen to twenty minutes.

3. Add water, pepper, sea salt, and broccoli sprouts. Cook on a simmer for twenty minutes.
4. Stir in quinoa and cook for ten minutes. Let cool for five minutes before stirring in olive oil.
5. Serve topped with basil leaves.

Chapter 5 Alkaline Diet-Accepted Snacks and Desserts

Avo Green Pea Spread
Ingredients:
Himalayan sea salt (1/4 teaspoon + 1/8 teaspoon)
Black pepper (1/8 teaspoon)
Chives/green onion, chopped finely (3 tablespoons + 1 teaspoon)
Green peas (2 cups)
Avocado, small, pitted, chopped roughly (1 piece)
Lime juice (2 ½ tablespoons)

Directions:
1. Place all ingredients in blender.
2. Process until well-mixed and smooth.
3. Enjoy.

Spinach Power Balls
Ingredients:
Wet mixture:
Lemon juice (1 tablespoon)
Garlic powder (1 teaspoon)
Sea salt (3/4 teaspoon)
Spinach leaves, organic (4 ½ cups)
Greek olives, pitted (1/3 cup)
Coconut yogurt (1 tablespoon)
Dry mixture:
Almonds, raw, ground (1/2 cup)
Almond flour (1/2 cup)
Brown rice, cooked (1 ¼ cups)

For serving:
Coconut yogurt

Directions:
1. Set oven at 360 degrees Fahrenheit to preheat.
2. Process all wet mixture ingredients in the blender. Pour into a large bowl.
3. Combine all dry mixture ingredients. Add to the wet mixture bowl and mix to form a dough-like mixture. Shape into 12 balls and arrange on a parchment-lined baking tray.
4. Bake for twenty-five minutes.
5. Serve with coconut yogurt.

Roasted Almonds
Ingredients:
Almonds, raw (2 cups)
Himalayan sea salt (1 teaspoon)
Olive oil (1/4 cup)

Directions:
1. Set oven at 275 degrees Fahrenheit to preheat.
2. Toss almonds with olive oil. Spread on an ungreased baking sheet.
3. Bake for twenty minutes. Sprinkle with sea salt and bake for another five minutes.
4. Let cool before serving.

Zucchini Chips
Ingredients:
Zucchinis, sliced w/ mandoline (6 pieces)
Sea salt (1/4 teaspoon)
Olive oil (1 teaspoon)

Directions:
1. Toss zucchini pieces with sea salt and olive oil.
2. Spread on parchment-lined cookie sheet.
3. Bake for fifteen minutes at 350 degrees Fahrenheit.

Lemony Roasted Artichokes
Ingredients:
Olive oil (1 ½ tablespoons + 1 ½ tablespoons)
Himalayan sea salt (1/4 teaspoon)
Black pepper, freshly ground (1/4 teaspoon)
Parsley, flat-leaf (1 tablespoon)
Globe artichoke, trimmed, sliced into wedges (1 piece)
Lemon juice, fresh (1/2 tablespoon)
Garlic cloves, unpeeled (6 pieces)
Lemon rind, cut into 2 strips (1/2 piece)

Directions:
1. Set oven at 480 degrees Fahrenheit.
2. Place lemon in a bowl filled with cold water (filtered/alkaline). Add the artichoke wedges and set aside.
3. Drain artichoke wedges and spread on the roasting tin. Add the garlic cloves and toss everything with olive oil (1 ½

tablespoons). After sprinkling with sea salt, roast for forty minutes, stirring halfway.
4. Add lemon rind strips to a saucepan filled with cold water (filtered/alkaline). Heat to boiling, then let simmer for five minutes. Drain, rinse, and roughly chop the boiled rind.
5. Let the roasted artichokes cool on a platter. Top with parsley.
6. Mash the roasted garlic cloves and boiled lemon rind. Mix with lemon juice and remaining olive oil (1 ½ tablespoons). Serve dip with the artichokes.

Guacamole and Mushroom Bites
Ingredients:
Olive oil (2 teaspoons)
Garlic clove, minced (1 piece)
Lime juice, fresh (2 tablespoons, divided)
Sea salt (1 pinch)
Pepper, ground (1 pinch)
Avocado, peeled, w/ pit removed (1 piece)
Cherry tomatoes, diced (3 pieces)
Cucumber, sliced (1 piece)
Mushrooms, drained (15 ounces)

Directions:
1. Combine mushrooms, half of the lime juice, and olive oil in a bowl. Add pepper and sea salt.
2. Mash the avocado, minced garlic, diced tomatoes, and remaining lime juice in

another bowl. Season with pepper and sea salt as well.
3. Spread cucumber pieces on serving tray. Add mushroom mixture on top of each cucumber piece. Finish by topping with guacamole and cherry tomatoes.

Delicious Cinnamon Carrot Sticks
Ingredients:
Salt (1 pinch)
Carrots, peeled (1 pound)
Cinnamon, ground (1 tablespoon)
Almond butter (1 tablespoon)

Directions:
1. Slice carrots into slender sticks. Steam for five minutes.
2. Toss carrots with remaining ingredients before placing in the boiler.
3. Cook on low for two minutes or until all carrot pieces are well-coated.

Beetroot Ravioli Snack
Ingredients:
Parsley, chopped finely (1 handful)
Red onion (1/4 piece)
Chives, chopped finely (1 ½ tablespoons)
Himalayan sea salt (1/4 teaspoon)
Black pepper (1/4 teaspoon)
Beetroots, large, peeled, sliced into rounds (2 pieces)
Lemon (1/2 piece)

Pine nuts, raw (1 cup)
Water, alkaline/filtered (1/2 cup)
Lemon juice (2 tablespoons)
Olive oil

Directions:
1. Process the pine nuts, water, onion, chives, parsley, and lemon juice in the blender until smooth.
2. Sprinkle pepper and sea salt over beetroot pieces.
3. Assemble raviolis by topping half of the beetroot rounds with pine nut cream and then covering with the remaining beetroot rounds.
4. Serve and enjoy.

Garlic Broccoli Roast
Ingredients:
Garlic cloves, fresh, sliced thinly (10 pieces)
Sea salt (1/4 teaspoon)
Broccoli, cut into 1-inch chunks (1 bunch)
Olive/coconut oil (3 tablespoons)
Black pepper (1/4 teaspoon)

Directions:
1. Set oven at 390 degrees Fahrenheit to preheat.
2. Toss broccoli and garlic with olive oil, pepper, and sea salt. Spread on ungreased baking sheet.
3. Roast for twenty to thirty minutes, turning halfway.

Stuffed Peppers and Tomatoes

Ingredients:

Garlic cloves, crushed (2 pieces)
Almonds, raw, chopped (3 tablespoons + 3 tablespoons)
Brown rice, cooked (75 grams)
Mint, chopped roughly (1 handful)
Green pepper (1 piece)
Yellow/red pepper (1 piece)
Tomatoes, ripe, large (2 pieces)
Onions, chopped (2 pieces)
Parsley, chopped roughly (1 handful)
Mixed herbs, fresh, chopped (1 tablespoon)
Celtic sea salt (1/4 teaspoon)
Black pepper, ground (1/4 teaspoon)
Olive oil (4 tablespoons)

Directions:

1. Set oven at 370 degrees Fahrenheit to preheat.
2. Carefully slice tomatoes in half and remove the pulp and seeds. Drain the tomato skins and roughly chop up the seeds and pulp.
3. Slice peppers in half; remove the seeds but leave the cores intact. Brush with olive oil (1 tablespoon) before baking for 15 minutes.
4. Place tomatoes in your oven-proof dish. Add the peppers and sprinkle with pepper and sea salt.
5. Cook the onions in remaining oil for five minutes. Stir in the almonds and cook for

another one minute. Turn off heat and mix in the cooked rice, mint, and parsley.
6. Fill the peppers and tomatoes with the rice mixture. Pour water (150 milliliters) around the stuffed peppers and tomatoes and bake for twenty minutes, uncovered. Top with almonds, drizzle with olive oil, and bake for another twenty minutes.
7. Serve topped with mixed herbs.

Tasty Sweet Potato Chips
Ingredients:
Sweet potato, large, peeled, cubed (3 pieces)
Himalayan sea salt (1/4 teaspoon)
Pepper, ground (1/4 teaspoon)
Olive oil (2 tablespoons)
Cayenne pepper (1/4 teaspoon)

Directions:
1. Set oven at 450 degrees Fahrenheit to preheat.
2. Lay sweet potato pieces on a foiled-lined tray and toss with a mixture of olive oil, cayenne pepper, and stevia. Season with pepper and sea salt.
3. Bake for eight minutes on each side.

Easy Pickled Cucumbers
Ingredients:
Sea salt (1 teaspoon)
Coriander, crushed (1 teaspoon)

Dill, fresh (1 tablespoon) or dill, dried (1 teaspoon)
Cucumbers, sliced w/ crinkle tool (1 cup)
Filtered water (1/2 cup)
Key lime juice, fresh (1 tablespoon)
Red pepper, crushed (1/2 teaspoon)

Directions:
1. Place all ingredients inside a glass jar.
2. Give jar a good shake.
3. Refrigerate for six to eight hours, shaking the mixture every hour.

Chocolate Pudding
Ingredients:
Orange zest (1 teaspoon)
Orange juice, freshly squeezed (1/2 cup)
Sea salt (1/8 teaspoon)
Vanilla bean, w/ seeds removed (1 piece)
Avocado, chopped roughly (1 cup)
Dates, pitted (1 cup)
Raw cacao powder (1/3 cup)

Directions:
1. Process all ingredients in the blender to form a smooth mixture.
2. Refrigerate for five hours.
3. Serve and enjoy.

Alkaline Energy Crackers
Ingredients:
Garlic clove, crushed (1 piece)

Cayenne pepper (1/2 teaspoon)
Salt (1/4 teaspoon)
Pepper, ground (1/4 teaspoon)
Water, filtered/alkaline (1 ¼ cups)
Chia seeds (1/2 cup)
Sesame seeds (1/2 cup)
Pumpkin seeds (1/2 cup)
Sunflower seeds (1/2 cup)

Directions:
1. Set oven at 300 degrees Fahrenheit to preheat.
2. Combine all ingredients. Let sit for ten minutes.
3. Spread mixture into an even layer on a parchment-lined baking tray. Bake for thirty minutes on each side.

Best Braccamole
Ingredients:
Hot sauce (1/8 teaspoon)
Avocado, peeled, pitted (1 piece)
Cherry tomatoes (1/2 cup)
Red onion, chopped finely (1/8 piece)
Broccoli, organic, raw, chopped, steamed (1 cup)
Lime juice, fresh (2 tablespoons)
Garlic clove, chopped roughly (1 piece)
Cumin (1/4 teaspoon)
Cilantro, chopped (3 tablespoons)

Directions:
1. Process broccoli, half of avocado, garlic, lime juice, and cumin in the blender until smooth.
2. Use a fork to mash remaining half of avocado before adding to the broccoli mixture. Add cilantro, pepper, sea salt, and tomatoes and mix well.
3. Refrigerate before serving.

Ginger Cookie Bites
Ingredients:
Brown rice syrup (2 tablespoons)
Medjool dates, pitted (4 pieces)
Cinnamon, ground (2 teaspoons)
Ginger, ground (3 teaspoons)
Almond butter (3 tablespoons)
Pine nuts, raw (1/4 cup)
Almonds, raw (1/4 cup)
Coconut oil (2 tablespoons)
Cardamom, ground (1 teaspoon)
Nutmeg, ground (1 pinch)
Millet, cooked (1 cup)

Directions:
1. Process dates, millet, almond butter, brown rice syrup, coconut oil, cinnamon, nutmeg, ginger, and cardamom in the blender until smooth.
2. Add the pine nuts and almonds and process until you have a slightly chunky mixture.

3. Shape mixture into cookie shapes and freeze for one hour.
4. Serve and enjoy.

Pine Nut Cream Cheese Spread
Ingredients:
Lemon juice, fresh (2 tablespoons)
Sea salt (1/2 teaspoon)
Pine nuts, raw (1 1/2 cups)
Garlic cloves (2 pieces)
Water, alkaline (1/4 cup)

Directions:
1. Place all ingredients in the blender.
2. Process until creamy and smooth.
3. Enjoy.

Oven-Baked Almond Cheese
Ingredients:
Coconut oil (1 tablespoon)
Garlic clove (1 piece)
Sea salt (1 1/2 teaspoons)
Almonds, raw (1 1/2 cups)
Lemon juice, fresh (1/4 cup)
Alkaline/filtered water (1/2 cup)
Olive oil (2 tablespoons)

Directions:
1. Process all ingredients in the blender until smooth.

2. Place mixture in a clean cheesecloth, set on a sieve placed over a bowl, and refrigerate overnight.
3. Transfer mixture into a greased dish (oven-proof). Bake for thirty-five to forty minutes at 350 degrees Fahrenheit.
4. Serve immediately.

Sweet Potato Brownies

Ingredients:
Himalayan sea salt (1 pinch)
Coconut oil, melted (1/4 cup)
Brown rice syrup (1/4 cup)
Sweet potato, medium, whole (1 piece)
Almonds, raw (2 cups)
Raw cacao powder (5 tablespoons)
Coconut flour (1 tablespoon)

Directions:
1. Chop sweet potatoes into two-inch cubes before boiling for fifteen to twenty minutes. Let cool.
2. Process almonds, sea salt, and raw cacao powder in the blender until well-combined. Add to a bowl filled with coconut flout, brown rice syrup, and coconut oil. Mix well.
3. Mash the cooled sweet potatoes and then fold into the almond mixture. Spread and press onto a parchment-lined pan. Freeze for one to two hours before serving.

Zucchini Flax Crackers
Ingredients:
Zucchini, pulped (1 cup)
Kale, organic, pulped (1/2 cup)
Flax seed, ground (2 tablespoons)
Sea salt (1/4 teaspoon)
Pepper, freshly ground (1/4 teaspoon)

Directions:
1. Combine all ingredients.
2. Shape mixture into crackers and set on the food dehydrator tray. Season with pepper and sea salt.
3. Dehydrate for six hours.
4. Serve and enjoy.

Marinated Zucchini Chips
Ingredients:
Zucchini, large, sliced (1 piece)
Marinade:
Cayenne (1/4 teaspoon)
Onion powder (2 ½ teaspoons)
Basil (1/2 teaspoon)
Lemon juice, fresh (4 tablespoons)
Olive oil (2 ½ tablespoons)
Paprika (1/2 teaspoon)
Celtic sea salt (1/2 teaspoon)
Oregano (1/2 teaspoon)

Directions:
1. Cut zucchini into thin slices.
2. Combine all marinade ingredients. Add zucchini slices and toss until well-coated.

3. Add zucchini pieces to dehydrator tray and dehydrate for fourteen to twenty hours.

Red Pepper and Almond Spread
Ingredients:
Olive oil (1/2 tablespoon)
Flax oil (1/2 tablespoon)
Cumin, ground (1/2 teaspoon)
Himalayan sea salt (1/4 teaspoon)
Black pepper (1/4 teaspoon)
Red bell pepper (1 piece)
Almonds, raw (1/2 cup)
Flaxseeds, ground (50 grams)

Directions:
1. Grill the red bell pepper to blacken the skin and easily peel it away.
2. Add red bell pepper to a blender filled with all other ingredients. Process until well-combined.
3. Serve and enjoy.

Green Peas Hummus
Ingredients:
Garlic clove, crushed (1 piece)
Sesame seeds (1 teaspoon)
Red chili (1 pinch)
Green peas, rinsed, drained (200 grams)
Lemon juice, fresh (2 teaspoons)
Basil leaves (1 handful)

Directions:
1. Add all ingredients to the blender.
2. Process until evenly mixed.
3. Serve and enjoy.

Pea and Broccoli Spread
Ingredients:
Olive oil (1/3 cup)
Celtic sea salt (1/2 teaspoon)
Mint, fresh (1 handful)
Coriander (3 sprigs)
Peas, steamed (2 cups)
Broccoli (1 cup)
Avocado (1/3 piece)
Garlic cloves (1 piece)
Lemon juice (2 tablespoons)
Lemon zest (1 teaspoon)

Directions:
1. Chop the broccoli, avocado, peas, mint, garlic, and coriander. Add to a blender filled with remaining ingredients.
2. Process until well-combined.
3. Serve with your favorite veggies.

Alkaline Granola Bars
Ingredients:
Sunflower seeds, raw (2 tablespoons)
Flax seeds (2 tablespoons)
Hemp seeds (2 tablespoons)
Stevia (1/4 cup)
Millet, toasted (1 ½ cups)

Almonds, raw, chopped roughly, toasted (1/2 cup)
Dates, pitted (1 ¼ cups)
Chia seeds (2 tablespoons)
Almond butter (1/4 cup)

Directions:
1. Process dates in the blender until dough-like in texture. Pour into a large bowl filled with the seeds, stevia, millet and almonds. Mix well.
2. Add almond butter to a saucepan heated on low. Once melted, add to the millet mixture. Mix everything well.
3. Place mixture in a parchment-lined dish (8x8). Cover with parchment and flatten until tightly packed. Freeze for thirty minutes.
4. Slice into 10 bars and serve.

Green Pea Patties
Ingredients:
Coconut aminos (1/2 cup)
Celtic sea salt (1 tablespoon)
Parsley, fresh (2 tablespoons)
Onion, chopped (1/2 cup)
Green peas (1 ½ cups)
Sunflower seeds (1 cup)
Garlic, minced (1 tablespoon)
Coriander, fresh, chopped (2 cups)
Lemon juice, fresh (1/2 cup)
Olive oil (1/2 cup)
Cumin (1 ½ teaspoons)

Directions:
1. Process all ingredients in the blender. Shape mixture into patties.
2. Set patties on a dehydrator tray lined with parchment. Dehydrate for three hours on one side. Flip patties and dehydrate for another five hours.

Spicy Herbed Flax Crackers
Ingredients:
Lime juice, fresh (1/4 cup)
Cumin (1 tablespoon)
Celtic/Himalayan sea salt (1 tablespoon)
Chili powder (1 pinch)
Sunflower seeds, soaked (1/2 cup)
Almonds, raw, soaked (1/2 cup)
Sundried tomatoes, soaked (1/4 cup)
Bell pepper, red, chopped (1 piece)
Coriander, fresh (1 tablespoon)
Basil, fresh (1 tablespoon)
Parsley, fresh (1 tablespoon)
Flaxseeds (1 cup)

Directions:
1. Process all ingredients in the food process or blender.
2. Spread mixture into an even, thin layer on a dehydrator tray lined with a silicone rubber mat. Dehydrate for two to three hours. Flip and dehydrate for another ten hours.

Tomato Pate
Ingredients:
Lime juice, fresh (1 tablespoon)
Basil, fresh, chopped (2 teaspoons)
Garlic clove, chopped roughly (1 piece)
Himalayan sea salt (1/4 teaspoon)
Sunflower seeds, soaked (1 cup)
Sundried tomatoes, soaked (1/3 cup)
Water, alkaline/filtered (2 tablespoons)
Red onion, diced finely (1 tablespoon)
Black pepper (1/4 teaspoon)

Directions:
1. Place all ingredients in the blender.
2. Process until smooth and creamy.
3. Serve and enjoy.

Decadent Avocado Chocolate Pudding
Ingredients:
Raw cacao (2 tablespoons)
Dates (3 pieces)
Sea salt (1 teaspoon)
Avocado (1 ½ pieces)
Coconut water (2/3 cup)
Vanilla (1 tablespoon)

Directions:
1. Fill the blender with all the ingredients.
2. Process at high speed until creamy in consistency.
3. Refrigerate for one hour before serving.

Mouthwatering Meltaway Balls
Ingredients:
Lemon juice, fresh (3/4 cup)
Vanilla (2 teaspoons)
Coconut oil (1/4 cup)
Almond flour (1 ½ cups)
Coconut flour (1/3 cup)
Himalayan sea salt (1/2 teaspoon)
Stevia (1 tablespoon)

Directions:
1. Process all ingredients in the blender until well-mixed.
2. Shape mixture into balls.
3. Refrigerate for fifteen minutes.
4. Serve and enjoy.

Coconut Lime Pana Cotta
Ingredients:
Stevia (3 tablespoons)
Lime zest (1 teaspoon)
Berries, chopped (1/4 cup)
Water, filtered (1/2 cup)
Coconut milk (1/2 cup)
Agar agar powder (1/2 teaspoon)
Lime juice, fresh (1 tablespoon)

Directions:
1. In a saucepan, mix agar agar powder and ¼ cup of filtered water. Let stand for five minutes.

2. In another saucepan, heat the coconut milk until warmed through.
3. Heat the agar agar mixture on low. Cook until boiling, then stir in remaining ingredients. Cook for another three to four minutes.
4. Pour into small bowls and let stand in the fridge for one hour.

Sea Salted Caramel Bars
Ingredients:
Base:
Medjool dates, soft (6 pieces)
Shredded coconut (1 ½ cups)
Cinnamon (1 pinch)
1st Layer:
Himalayan sea salt (1 pinch)
Coconut oil (1 tablespoon)
Coconut aminos (1/2 cup)
Vanilla (1/4 teaspoon)
Coconut cream (1/2 cup)
Medjool dates (3 pieces)
Coconut syrup (2 tablespoons)
2nd Layer:
Vanilla (1/4 teaspoon)
Cinnamon (1 pinch)
Coconut syrup (1 tablespoon)
Coconut oil (3 tablespoons)
Raw cacao powder (1 tablespoon)

Directions:
1. Process all base ingredients in the blender. Spread onto a baking tin.

2. Blend the 1st layer ingredients and spread onto the base.
3. Blend the 2nd layer ingredients and spread on top of the 1st layer.
4. Refrigerate for one hour before serving.

Carrot Cake Bites
Ingredients:
Almonds, raw (40 grams)
Cinnamon (1 ½ teaspoons)
Orange juice (2 teaspoons)
Orange zest (1 teaspoon)
Sunflower seeds (1/2 cup)
Millet (1 cup)
Medjool dates, pitted (5 pieces)
Carrots, grated (180 grams)
Raisins (1/4 cup)
Coconut oil (1 tablespoon)
Desiccated coconut, unsweetened (3 tablespoons)

Directions:
1. Place all ingredients, save for the desiccated coconut, in the blender and proess until well-combined.
2. Shape the mixture into balls.
3. Cover with desiccated coconut and serve.

Lemon, Coconut and Pine Nut Balls
Ingredients:
Chia seeds (2 tablespoons)
Lemon (1 piece)

Sea salt (1/2 teaspoon)
Vanilla (2 teaspoons)
Desiccated coconut, unsweetened (1/2 cup)
Medjool dates, pitted (180 grams)
Pine nuts, raw (1 ¼ cups)
Pea protein powder, vegan/alkaline, neutral flavored (1/2 cup)
To serve:
Desiccated coconut, unsweetened (1/2 cup)

Directions:
1. Process all ingredients in the blender.
2. Mold into balls and sprinkle all over with desiccated coconut.
3. Refrigerate for one hour.
4. Enjoy.

Matcha Almond Balls
Ingredients:
Shredded coconut, unsweetened (1/4 cup)
Matcha protein powder, vegan/alkaline (2 teaspoons)
Coconut oil (1 tablespoon)
Almonds, raw, whole (3/4 cup)
Pine nuts, raw, shelled (1/4 cup)
Medjool dates, pitted (12 pieces)
Almonds, raw, chopped (1/4 cup)

Directions:
1. Put all ingredients in the blender.
2. Process until evenly combined.
3. Roll mixture into balls.

4. Let sit in the fridge for fifteen minutes before serving.

Apricot Almond Balls
Ingredients:
Apricots, dried, chopped roughly (1 cup)
Coconut butter (1 cup + 2 tablespoons)
Almonds, raw (1/2 cup)
Desiccated coconut, unsweetened (2 tablespoons)

Directions:
1. Add all ingredients to the food processor.
2. Process until well-mixed.
3. Shape into balls and set on a tray.
4. Let bon bons set in the refrigerator within thirty minutes.

Chewy Chocolate Bon Bons
Ingredients:
Raw cacao powder (2 tablespoons)
Stevia (1 tablespoon)
Sea salt (1 pinch)
Desiccated coconut, unsweetened (1 cup)
Almonds, raw, ground (1/2 cup)
Dates, pitted (1 cup)

Directions:
1. Fill the food processor with all ingredients.
2. Blitz until everything is well-combined.

3. Form the mixture into small balls.
4. Let chill in the fridge for an hour.
5. Serve and enjoy.

Pecan Pie Bites
Ingredients:
Millet (1/2 cup)
Cinnamon (1 teaspoon)
Stevia (2 tablespoons)
Medjool dates, pitted (2 cups)
Pumpkin seeds (1 ½ cups)

Directions:
1. Add all ingredients to the food processor. Blitz until well-mixed.
2. Shape mixture into 25 balls.
3. Let the balls firm up in the refrigerator for twenty minutes.
4. Serve and enjoy.

Amazing Almond Balls
Ingredients:
Sea salt (1/4 teaspoon)
Vanilla (1/2 teaspoon)
Almond milk, unsweetened (2 tablespoons)
Dates, pitted (2 cups)
Almonds, raw (2 cups)
Cocoa powder, unsweetened (1/4 cup)
Coconut flakes, unsweetened (3/4 cup)

Directions:
1. Place all ingredients in the food processor.
2. Process until you have an evenly combined mixture.
3. Refrigerate for one hour.
4. Serve and enjoy.

Chia Coconut Bites
Ingredients:
Medjool dates, pitted (4 pieces)
Raw cacao powder (1/3 cup)
Pine nuts, raw (1/3 cup)
Almonds, raw (1/4 cup)
Almond meal (1 cup)
Shredded coconut, unsweetened (1/2 cup)
Coconut oil (1/3 cup)
Chia seeds (1 tablespoon)

Directions:
1. Process all ingredients in the blender until evenly mixed.
2. Roll into small balls.
3. Serve immediately.

Key Lime Pie Bites
Ingredients:
Lime zest (2 tablespoons)
Lime juice, fresh (3 tablespoons)
Sea salt (1 pinch)
Medjool dates, pitted (3/4 cup)
Pine nuts, raw (1 cup)
Shredded coconut, unsweetened (1/2 cup)

Directions:
1. Put all ingredients in the blender and process until smooth.
2. Mold mixture into balls.
3. Let sit in the fridge for one hour before serving.

Papaya Boats
Ingredients:
Blueberries (1/4 cup)
Almonds, raw, slivered (2 tablespoons)
Chia seeds (1 tablespoon)
Hemp seeds, hulled (1/2 tablespoon)
Papaya, medium, w/ flesh scooped out (1 piece)
Bananas, , large, frozen (2 pieces)
Coconut yogurt (1 cup)
Kiwi, medium (1 piece)
Sweet cherry, raw, halved, pitted (1/2 cup)
Sunflower seeds (1 tablespoon)

Directions:
1. Scoop out the flesh from the papaya.
2. Process frozen bananas in the blender until creamy.
3. Fill papaya shells with banana ice cream, then top with all other ingredients.
4. Serve and enjoy.

Apple and Pear Crumble
Ingredients:
Nutmeg (1/2 teaspoon)

Millet (1/4 cup)
Almonds, raw, chopped (1/4 cup)
Coconut oil (1 tablespoon)
Green apple, chopped (1 piece)
Pear, sliced (1 piece)
Cinnamon (1 teaspoon)

Directions:

1. Add coconut oil to a saucepan heated on medium.
2. Stir in pears, apple slices, nutmeg, and cinnamon. Cook for five minutes.
3. Ladle into 2 bowls. Serve topped with millet, almonds, and extra cinnamon.

Conclusion

I'd like to thank you and congratulate you for transiting my lines from start to finish.

I hope this book was able to help you see how important it is to be mindful about what you eat, especially in terms of keeping your blood and body alkaline and ensuring that you are not feeding it unnecessary, unhealthy, and harmful acid-forming foods. I hope this book also helps you realize that, far from limiting yourself to a joyless way of eating, the alkaline diet actually gives you the freedom to enjoy different foods without putting your health on the line.

The next step is to slowly but surely get on the alkaline diet track. Remember to enjoy the journey while you reap all of the health benefits.

I wish you the best of luck!

www.ingramcontent.com/pod-product-compliance
Lightning Source LLC
Chambersburg PA
CBHW070254010526
44107CB00056B/2455